William Fordyce

A review of the venereal disease, and its remedies

William Fordyce

A review of the venereal disease, and its remedies

ISBN/EAN: 9783337733544

Printed in Europe, USA, Canada, Australia, Japan

Cover: Foto ©ninafisch / pixelio.de

More available books at **www.hansebooks.com**

A
REVIEW

OF THE

VENEREAL DISEASE.

[Price Three Shillings.]

A REVIEW

OF THE

VENEREAL DISEASE,

AND

ITS REMEDIES.

BY WILLIAM FORDYCE,
M.D. BY ROYAL MANDATE.

THE FOURTH EDITION,

WITH CONSIDERABLE

ADDITIONS, AND AN APPENDIX.

LONDON:
Printed by T. SPILSBURY, Snow Hill,
For T. CADELL, in the Strand;
And Sold by J. MURRAY, in Fleet-Street; and
W. DAVENHILL, in Cornhill.

MDCCLXXVIII.

TO

SIR WILLIAM DUNCAN BART.

THE FOLLOWING REVIEW

IS

WITH THE HIGHEST ESTEEM

FOR HIS MEDICAL TALENTS

AND

THE SINCEREST RESPECT

FOR HIS PERSONAL CHARACTER

INSCRIBED

BY THE AUTHOR.

	Pag.
INTRODUCTION - - - - -	1.

SECT. I.
Opinions of the most celebrated writers on this disease - - - - - - - - 3

SECT. II.
On the different species of the gonorrhœa - 22

SECT. III.
Necessary observations - - - - - - 28

SECT. IV.
On the cure of the gonorrhœa - - - - 33

SECT. V.
Remarks on the first and second species - - 40

SECT. VI.
General remarks - - - - - - - - 42

SECT. VII.
Of the swelled testicle - - - - - - 44

SECT. VIII.
Of gleets - - - - - - - - - 51

SECT.

	Pag.
SECT. IX.	
Of bougies - - - - - - - - - -	58
SECT. X.	
Of buboes - - - - - - - - - -	62
SECT. XI.	
Of chancres - - - - - - - - -	67
SECT. XII.	
Of other pocky symptoms - - - - - -	70
SECT. XIII.	
Necessary remarks on the disease - - -	76
SECT. XIV.	
A problem - - - - - - - - - -	81
SECT. XV.	
Of mercury and its preparations - - - -	82
SECT. XVI.	
On the present state of the pox - - - -	105
APPENDIX - - - - - - -	107

A REVIEW

OF THE

VENEREAL DISEASE, &c.

INTRODUCTION.

SO much has been written, both by surgeons and physicians, concerning the Venereal Disease, and so much is supposed to be known by every quack, and apothecary's apprentice, about its treatment; that it may be thought presumptuous, or at least superfluous, to say more upon the subject. But nothing certainly can be so effectual an obstruction to the progress of knowledge in general, as an opinion

opinion that no room is left for farther improvement. Long and large experience has convinced me, that this particular branch does ſtill admit of a great deal; and the dreadful conſequences ariſing from the groſs ignorance of many practitioners, as well as from the ſhameful impoſitions of not a few, are every day but too apparent. What increaſes the miſchief exceedingly, is the inattention of the patients themſelves to their own health, no leſs than their indifference about the welfare of their poſterity. On theſe accounts, I find myſelf prompted to communicate my obſervations on this diſeaſe, in hopes of rendering it leſs deſtructive to mankind, by enabling each individual, who unhappily labours under it, to judge whether he is in ſkilful and honeſt hands, or the contrary.

Whatever deference is due to writers of reputation, in thoſe particular caſes, where

the

the rules by them laid down for the management of diseases remain to this day the best standard of practice; that very deference will prove a false guide, if extended to subjects where the lights, which they had acquired, were in reality but the dawn of what is now more fully known. It must therefore be of consequence to guard beginners in the healing art against an implicit reliance even on the greatest professors.

Warwick-street, Westminster,
March 31, 1777.

SECTION I.

Opinions of the most celebrated writers on this disease.

DR. Sydenham has justly acquired the highest rank in the profession of physic; and to his capacity, equalled only by his candour, I bow with respect. But that

that great man, it is very certain, has advanced pofitions on this point, which do not well agree with our prefent knowledge of it. According to him, the cure of a clap depends wholly on purging medicines, by which the peccant humour is difcharged, or a diverfion is made of the natural juices, that might otherwife feed the difeafe. Any purgative long perfevered in, he believes, will be fuccefsful, but efpecially the more draftic kinds; and he particularly recommends a form of that fort to be taken daily, for the firft twelve or fourteen days, or more. Neverthelefs, fo far as I have had opportunities of obferving, I muft be of opinion, that either in delicate, or irritable habits, nothing tends fo directly to keep up the cordee, to bring on ftrangury and fever, or to produce fwelled tefticles, as draftic and daily purging, though even of the mercurial kind. But who would not guard, if pof-
fible,

sible, against every one of these symptoms? The last in particular, that of swelled testicles, seems to me in its consequences the most formidable that can befall the patient, and the most troublesome to the practitioner; whether you speak of his reputation which is concerned to prevent, or of the skill which is required to conquer it, and to put a stop to the terrible inroads it makes on the constitution.

To proceed with our admired author; he does not prescribe bleeding, even in sanguine temperaments, and where the complaint is obstinate, till after a month's purging; "lest," says he, "it should "throw the disease into the habit." But now, if, during this purgation for a month, the strangury, continual cordee, watchfulness, or fever, occasioned by so heating a method of cure, even in spite of a severe course of diet; if these evils, I say, are
not

not alleviated by bleeding, opiates, and abstinence from meat, which last he does not require, what are the consequences? A fever supervenes, by which the flow of the virulent matter from the urethra is stopt, and the disease is blended with the constitution; or there is produced in the testicles a swelling, of which the resolution is tedious, difficult, and full of danger.

Another position of this celebrated writer is, that purging is every thing here, and that in this disease, if in any, it may be said, " He cures well who " cleanses well." On such authority, who would not be tempted to trust to purging alone, and even to carry it to the utmost? How often have I done so, till I was taught better, and emboldened by experience to set aside the authority of even a Sydenham; by following whom, in this instance, I had the mortification to find my patients declining daily, and

groaning

groaning under a tedious gleet without any relief!

He adds indeed, " If the method above " mentioned does not fucceed in ftopping " the gonorrhœa, it may be done more " effectually by a ftrong purge; or, if " that fhould likewife fail, by two or " three dofes of turpeth mineral at proper " intervals, or elfe by a large dofe of ca- " lomel twice a week." All thefe however I muft in general difapprove, as fcarcely fuited to any but the moft robuft conftitutions.

After this he has recourfe to turpentine medicines, and the drying balfams; but without fpecifying fufficiently when they may be ufed with fafety, notwithftanding he feems fo well aware of the rifk the patient runs of falling into a confirmed pox, from the peccant humours not being properly carried off by purgatives, in conftitutions where there is an antipathy

pathy to thefe, or a difficulty of being purged.

As to his notion that the hardnefs in the prepuce, or the ulceration brought upon that part, or under it, is to be cured by fomentations, and mucilaginous or oily applications alone, or even by the mercurial preparation of precipitate mixed with a foftening ointment; I muft needs fay, that I do not find it correfpond with fact, having feen poxes often fuperinduced by this laft application; I mean, where the antivenereal courfe has not been firft regularly purfued. In that cafe, indeed, the method I fpeak of will foften the præputium, and enable the patient to return it; or the fame thing may be effected by the leaden cannula contrived and recommended by Fallopius, to which I have been frequently forced to have recourfe, when all the ulcers had difappeared.

With

With regard to the treatment of the swelled testicle; Dr. Sydenham does not give the least hint, that mercurial applications, or preparations, are often necessary to secure the patient from the pocky consequences of inflammations which happen frequently in that tender part.

But to conclude the strictures which justice to my subject has obliged me, however unwilling, to make on this truly great man; the principal objection to his method of treating the confirmed pox is his trusting for the cure to so small a quantity of the quicksilver rubbed on at first to raise a salivation, and his depending on alteratives afterwards given inwardly to keep it up: for I doubt not of being able to demonstrate in the proper place, that the security does not arise from the salivation, so much as from the quantity of quicksilver necessary to extinguish the symptoms.

C. Dr.

Dr. Boerhaave, after thirty six years close attention to the venereal disease, acknowledges, that, in a number of cases, he was still uncertain about the best method of treating it; and that the least circumstance mismanaged, or overlooked, was productive of complaints which he could not conquer.

After so candid an acknowledgement, may I not hope to be forgiven by the Boerhaavian school, justly respectable for having bred many who are now among the brightest ornaments of their profession, if I take the liberty to dispute several of that great man's opinions in relation to this disease; since it cannot seem strange, that the experience of thirty six years more, which have elapsed from the time he made the observation above mentioned, should have thrown such light on some particulars, as shews him to have been mistaken on a subject which by his own confession he found so difficult?

I begin with obferving, that his maxim of mercurial medicines being never neceffary in his firft fpecies of gonorrhœa, does not hold univerfally, it being certain that the pox has taken place, and been communicated to the wife, after the moft regular treatment upon his plan; probably indeed owing to the patient's having contracted this firft fpecies from a woman who was poxed.

In his fecond fpecies of the gonorrhœa, attentive obfervers muft have often feen the difeafe creep into the inguinal glands, during a courfe of brifk purging, accompanied with an antiphlogiftic regimen, for two whole months, although the running has not received the leaft check whatfoever.

With refpect to his third fpecies, where the complaint affects Cowper's glands of the urethra, he remarks that the fuccefs of the cure depends entirely on the whole of the infectious matter flowing off by means of the discharge; but he does not specify when mercurials are to be used, though he observes very justly, that the severe remedy of a salivation becomes here often necessary.

To his doctrine concerning the fourth species, where the prostate gland is affected, I should have no objection, as he recommends a salivation at once; provided he gave any caution about the impropriety of trusting to the purging course mixed with mercurials, by which the effects of mercury on the disease are always weakened; or provided he described the powers which belong to decoctions of sarsa, or balsamic drinks.

As to his fifth and last sort of gonorrhœa, where Morgagni's glands, and the seminal vesicles, &c. are affected, we must necessarily disapprove of his resting the patient's relief from this miserable state

on

on plasters, ointments, fomentations, poultices, the knife, the sweating box, diet drinks, abstinence, and severe salivations; without recommending, what we have generally found necessary in such a case, the use of mercurial ointment so moderately applied as not to break down the habit, or of Peruvian bark, open air, milk diet, and the soft decoctions.

We come now to his general maxims for the cure of a confirmed pox. This, he tells us, consists in drawing off all the fat of the body, even to the last particle; in which fat, according to his theory, the whole poison of the venereal malady is lodged. " For," continues he, " if
" the least particle remains, there is rea-
" son to fear a relapse; so that, unless
" the oils of the body, and this poi-
" son concreted in them, are entirely
" dissolved, and purged off, you can ne-
" ver

" ver (if the difease is inveterate) have a
" radical cure, but only the appearance
" of one, such as you will repent your
" having trusted to, very heartily. Now
" the effects here required are to be pro-
" duced by mercury; on whose action
" however you are not to rely, unless
" you reduce all the fat humours into
" water, expel them completely, and
" with them wash off entirely the ve-
" nereal poison." What is the infer-
ence? " That, in order to be properly
" cured of the pox, the patient must be
" fed on the leanest foods, kept in a
" great and continued heat, reduced to
" the paleness of a corpse; in a word,
" totally emaciated, and the cure pro-
" tracted, till he has got rid of all his old
" juices. If this counsel is not faithfully
" followed in curing him; and if, after
" you have cured him, you do not re-
" strain him, for a month or two longer,
" from

" from fat things of the putrefcent kind;
" you will have caufe to regret your
" having fubjected him in vain to the
" torture of fo fevere a courfe, fince there
" will be ftill fome relics of the difeafe
" lurking in the body, and buried there
" only for a time, to rife again with new
" ftrength and violence."

On reading, many years ago, the above theory of this eminent phyfiologift, I concluded from fo high an authority, that the difeafe could not be cured radically by any other method, and accordingly fet about treating the more ftubborn cafes in his way; till I difcovered that, notwithftanding the firmeft adherence to it, there frequently remained in the groins fuch obftinate and ill looking fores, as were not to be healed, till the natural balfam of the blood* was reftored by freer living,

by

* By the natural balfam of the blood being reftored, I would be underftood to mean, fuch a ftate

of

by fresh air, and a fuller habit. I likewise found, that the disease was only hid by this lowering plan, and broke out afresh upon the change to a plentiful diet. Neither indeed could it be well expected, that, in a country like this, your patients would submit to be starved, while their companions in the same situation were recovering daily by following a reasonable regimen.

He likewise urges the necessity of the same severe treatment, where the disease lies out of the course of circulation, among the bones, and therefore out of the reach of mercury. In that case, he allows his patient nothing but biscuit and raisins for food, with decoctions of guaiacum for drink; whereas, in our days, even when mercury fails, strong decoctions of juices as that which the disease, or the method of treatment, had destroyed, and which, till it is restored, not only prevents the recovery of strength, but the cure of the sores.

tions of sarsaparilla, without confinement or any particular regimen, produce, as we have proved elsewhere, a speedy, safe, and pleasant cure.* I have the most evident proofs that small exfoliations, not extending so far as the sutures which mark the boundaries of the small bones of the face, are thrown off by strong decoctions of sarsa; though this fact is very positively contradicted by our illustrious author.

The writer on this subject, who, of all that have yet treated it, seems beyond comparison to have understood it best, is Dr. Astruc. If the following short remarks on his work are found justified by facts, the candid reader will, I trust, forgive a freedom, which nothing but those facts could have induced me to take with so able a professor.

His notion that a gonorrhœa never terminates in a pox, provided the matter loaded

---

* See the Appendix.

loaded with the venereal contagion is freely and copiously discharged, tends to prevent the attention that is necessary for eradicating the whole infection; since we see every day, in many obstinate gonorrhœas, the worst consequences arising from the least neglect in prosecuting the antivenereal course, by mercury alone, or combined with sarsa, as appears to be indicated, to its full extent.

Nor does he seem to inculcate, with sufficient force, the necessity of employing mercurials, as soon as the double infection is discovered; neither can I find, that, in treating the gonorrhœa, he has determined to what extent they must be used for curing effectually its pocky attendants.

He seems not sufficiently aware of the risk the patient runs of getting poxed by strengthening and astringent medicines. But perhaps the French temperament and climate

climate may make a more material difference in the difeafe, and the effects of its remedies, than I have had accefs to obferve in this country.

Towards the end of his work, he has given us the hiftory of particular fymptoms and relics of this difeafe, that no plan with which he was acquainted could remove; fuch as certain fwellings in the tefticles which do not yield to the hydrargyrofis, diftortion of the penis, nodes, ganglions, tubercles, exoftofes, gummata, cancerous appearances, and old venereal fores, ulcers in the womb, &c. Yet we know affuredly, that all thefe may be cured by fome kinds of mineral waters, oranges, lemons, or other antifcorbutics, ftrong decoctions of farfa, and hemlock, outwardly and inwardly applied.

If upon the faireft trials, frequently repeated, I had, in all or in moft venereal cafes, found fuccefs from the folution of of corrosive sublimate, formerly used in this country;* ushered in afresh by such a master in medicine as Baron Van Swieten, and supported by his disciples at Vienna, and elsewhere,† with the evidence of innumerable cures registered in their hospitals‡ as performed by it; I should in that case have probably saved the world and myself the trouble of these sheets, whereof one main intention is, if possible, to put a stop, in these kingdoms, to the practice of relying on this corrosive medicine for the cure of almost every venereal complaint, however serious, and however much the object of the more momentous, and adequate antidote, mercurial ointment.

Whether its failure in my own experience, or under the careful management of many gentlemen in the profession, of my acquaintance, was owing to the nature

* Turner.
† Medical Essays of London.
‡ Locker.

ture of our climate, or to the state of the juices occasioned by so much animal food, or to the want of sufficient mercurial momentum in so small a quantity of the medicine as is generally used, I will not take upon me to say: but I am apt to believe, that by continuing to prefer the mercurial ointment to any of the preparations of mercury, I shall be frequently employed to complete, by inunction, that cure which others have attempted unsuccessfully with this now so fashionable medicine; of which I can affirm with certainty, that it failed very often in the British hospitals in Germany, as well as in the Isle of Wight, during the last war; and that it has done infinite mischief in this metropolis, under as many quackish names as there are advertisements in the news papers for the cure of the complaint.

From these few observations on what is advanced by some of the most celebrated

brated writers on this subject, I apprehend it appears, that the characteristics of the venereal disease, the nature of the remedies, and the fittest time of applying them, have not hitherto been generally understood; and therefore it is hoped the present attempt will not be deemed unnecessary. I am sure my end will be gained, if, by communicating information to some, and calling forth the experience of others, in so important a branch of the healing art, I may contribute any thing to the welfare of mankind.

SECTION II.

On the different species of the gonorrhœa.

THE period at which the venereal infection was brought from the West Indies into Europe is sufficiently ascertained, and the rapidity with which,

under

under different shapes, it soon after spread over the rest of the world, is commonly known. Without dwelling on circumstances so little interesting at this time, we will go on to trace the disease from its simplest appearances to its more complicated forms, and endeavour to establish such rules as shall at once determine its peculiar qualities, and point out the remedies, together with the regimen, requisite for the cure of its various stages.

It has been frequently asserted, that the division of the clap and pox into their different species is of little or no use. But if it is not known how far the disease has got into the genitals in the gonorrhœa, or into the habit in the lues venerea, I see not how the indications of cure can be so clearly discovered. If therefore we can make the division in question sufficiently intelligible to a sensible reader, though no anatomist, and, by ascertaining

the

the exact state of the distemper, can explain its proper treatment through its several stages, we shall have the pleasure of contributing to the comfort of every one who wishes to know whether he has obtained a complete cure, or if not, whether he is in the way to it.

A man in perfect health passes, by his urethra, urine and semen only, or perhaps now and then a little of that transparent mucus which lubricates the passage. The parts composing this passage, continued all the way up to the neck of the bladder, are the general seat of the gonorrhœa. If by manustupration, or early venery, he has weakened the seminal organs, he then often passes the seed before it is properly concocted or exalted, which debilitates the whole body, but more particularly the nervous system. This is called Tabes Dorsalis; an evil more dreadful in its consequences than the most virulent gonorrhœa,

norrhœa, and often producing tremors, palsies, melancholy, and madness. 'Tali tabe laborantes cœlibes vivant, nisi prius hæredes gignendi facultatem experti sint, ne nihil præter nothos et ingentem miseriam matrimonium sequatur.' I write as a physician, not as a casuist. Of this gonorrhœa we profess not to speak.

The most simple species of gonorrhœa, contracted by infection, is discerned by a discharge from the urethra, marking the linen with an ichorous kind of stain; in the middle of which there is commonly perceived a yellow or greenish coloured pus, about the size of a pin's head, together with, now and then, a single drop of the same sort lodged in the point of the urethra; and this attended with a scalding heat in the water, but without cordee, or any other violent symptom.

When, some days after the knowledge of a person infected, there appears an inflammation

flammation on the glans penis, with an oozing of matter from behind the nut, from the internal surface of the prepuce, or from the glans penis, but without ulceration, or any discharge from the urethra itself, and, on being touched by the urine, conveying the same sort of sensation which we call heat of water; this may be styled the second species of gonorrhœa.

When, on pressing the nut at any time, especially in the morning, there issues from the urethra a quantity of purulent matter, which seems to come from the body of the gland, or not farther back than about an inch from the orifice of the urethra; I would call this the third species. As it is the most common sort of any, so it is usually of long continuance.

When a plentiful discharge of matter flows into the whole cavity of the urethra,

and

and is supposed to have affected Cowper's glands, I would term it the fourth species of gonorrhœa.

In the fifth, the matter comes all the way from the neck of the bladder, and in very large quantities, attended with continual difficulty in making water, a fetid smell, and imposthumations outwardly on the perinæum, and ad anum.

If all these symptoms are advanced a stage higher, so as to affect the seminal vesicles, and to produce incontinency of water, or an incapacity of retaining the seed, it has been considered by some authors, as another, and the last species of gonorrhœa.

To me, it appears, that this sort, and the two immediately preceding, may be properly considered as pocky appearances, and ought certainly at once to be treated as such, since they will not yield to any medicine merely antiphlogistic.

Having thus described the different species of gonorrhœa, so as to enable any patient of ordinary understanding, to discover with exactness the stage of his distemper, I now proceed to point out the cure, after premising some observations, partly for the sake of preventing mistakes, and partly for paving the way to what shall follow.

SECTION III.

Necessary observations.

IN the first place, it is but fair to acknowledge, that where there is virulence in the gonorrhœa, our art cannot cure it speedily, and effectually, at the same time. Therefore the patient should not expect, nor the physician promise it. Unless the severest regimen is observed, it will often run out to two or three months, and in some cases to five or six.

In the next place, I muſt take the liberty to ſay, that the impropriety of eſtabliſhing infallible maxims never appeared more evident, than in the principal one which has been ſo frequently laid down on this ſubject; namely, that a large and continued running, kept up either by medicines, or by other proper methods, is the greateſt preſervative againſt a clap's becoming a confirmed pox; for, if the clap be of a bad ſort, it will in many caſes become a pox, by truſting to that very running; whereas, by the ſeaſonable interpoſition of mercury, the cure might be diſpatched time enough to avoid ſo diſagreeable an event. There are many people indeed, who, from an apprehenſion of mercury's producing pernicious effects on the conſtitution, will ſcarcely conſent to the uſe of it at all in what they call a clap. It will afterwards appear how ill grounded their fears are on this head.

The maxim above mentioned is, I confess, of real use, when it supersedes the necessity of employing astringents or injections, till there has been time given to remove the virulence, or when it prevents confiding in those whose boasted expeditious methods of treatment are calculated to ruin, not to save.

For my own part, I hold it as a principle, never to use either astringents, injections, or balsamics,* but in cases of extremity; nor even then, till I have, by a course of mercurial inunctions, provided against all the ill consequences of the disease, (supposing it to prove obstinate, and the running to continue discoloured) as well

---

* It were to be wished, that we could ascertain the exact period when balsamic medicines might be adopted with safety; as perhaps there are constitutions which would admit of their use much earlier than cautious practitioners generally imagine; while there are other habits, where their too precipitate application would extend the gonorrhœa to a dreadful length.

well as against any retention of morbid matter, by promoting in every possible way a free discharge for a proper time; and let me add, not till I have likewise tried, without effect, every method to restore the tone both of the part, and of the habit, in the manner that will be hereafter explained.

To brisk purgatives in this distemper I am utterly averse; and the gentler ones I am for using more rarely than is commonly practised. In truth, I generally suspect long continued discharges, as tending to produce a pox, or at least obstructions of the urethra, which last are not curable by topical applications alone.

During the whole course of a virulent gonorrhœa, there is danger of its being carried into the habit, by every thing that stops the discharge before the infection is removed. The discharge will be stopt by hurried walks, or violent exercise of any

any kind, especially on horseback; or by strong and drastic purges, whether common or mercurial, or by catching cold, or a fever fit, while under a purging course.

It deserves particular notice, that every thing promoting erections of the penis increases inflammation, sends the infection further back into the urethra, keeps up the disease, and often subjects the patient to all the inconveniences of a fresh antiphlogistic regimen for two or three weeks, in the same manner as if the cure was but just begun. Among the causes of such erections, may be reckoned chiefly a turtle feast,* a fish diet, hearty dinners, onions,

---

* I have not only often seen the disease recur, with all the symptoms of its first stage, in consequence of a turtle feast; but have once known a running, with inflammation, brought on by the same means, in a sober married man, who had been free from infection for many years: at least I could not trace it to any other source.

onions, spiceries,* high-seasoned foods of every sort, fermented liquors, hot suppers, women's company, and libidinous conversation.

If ever a strict attention to regimen is necessary in any disease, it is certainly in this, where the infection is recalled into the habit by every deviation in point of diet, or of exercise.

SECTION IV.

On the cure of the gonorrhœa.

THE generality of authors are agreed, that purging is the remedy for the gonorrhœa, as is salivation for a confirmed pox:

---

* I am informed by a friend lately arrived from the islands of Bourbon, that, having one day put a parcel of the Cayenne pepper in a handkerchief round his waist, his black servant told him, it would give him the clap. He had not seen a woman for eight months before. The prophecy was fulfilled in a day or two; and

pox: but it has not been explained with sufficient exactness, when the first cannot answer, any more than why the last often fails; nor whence proceeds the inefficacy in the former case, or what resources in both cases are still left.

If the procuring from two to four stools every other day, for the first fourteen days, and the same number every third day during the second fourteen days, does not considerably diminish the running, or change the yellow or yellowish-green matter into a discharge more seminal, ropy, and diluted in its colour; I should not hesitate in such a circumstance, even though the cordee or heat of urine were not removed, (and they will sometimes remain as at first) to apply such a preparation

and he found it necessary to be cured in the common way, by the advice of a surgeon there, who said it was a very usual effect of that spice in those islands. I mention this only as matter of curiosity, and not as part of my creed, though this has been alledged.

ration of mercury, more early in the difeafe, as I thought fafeft, and fit to be ufed in the largeft quantity. What that is, will be determined afterwards.

If the form of pills is preferred by the patient to half an ounce or more of falts and manna, (of each equal parts) then from ten to fifteen grains of jalap root, with as much nitre, mixed up into pills of the common fize, will probably be a proper quantity for producing the defired effect.

Or, if the form of an electuary is yet more agreeable, the following, which I would call the Elect. Diafenæ, will anfwer every purpofe that is to be obtained by purging.

 R. Elect. lenitiv. drach. vi.
  Pulv. e tragacanth. comp. unc. fs.
  ——— fol. fenæ drach. ii.
  ——— radic. jalap. drach. ifs.
  Syrup. rofar. folutiv. q. f. fiat electarium;
   cujus capiat q. n. m. majoris alterna vel
   tertia nocte, vel pro re nata.

If instead of such a course you purge daily, what is the consequence? You keep up a continual irritation on the bladder, by the tenesmus attending frequent purging, and an inclination to make water, or a stimulus all along the urethra, where the disease first lodges; than which nothing is more likely to prolong the inflammation, or to provoke a gleet. Now all this is prevented by gentle physic, taken every second or third day only.

It is a common practice to be perpetually diluting with large quantities of small drinks, ptisans with nitre, &c. When the pain in making water is not extreme, a moderate quantity of softening liquors, such as milk and water, water gruel, or linseed tea, answers the purpose much better, and flows off with less trouble, and fewer calls on the patient. An attention to this circumstance will, besides preventing much pain, forward the cure not a little. It

It is acknowledged, that, in very irritable, or spasmodic habits, gum arabic, and syrup of white poppies, are always useful, and sometimes necessary.

As to nitre, and diuretics in general, my objection to them is not answered by their antiphlogistic effects, while the same effects can be produced by diluent and softening drinks, or by bleeding, and abstinence from flesh, and from wine, spirits, or fermented liquors of any sort; and, above all the rest, by repose. By repose, I mean a sedentary life during the cure, or at least slow motion, either on foot, or in an easy carriage, and off the streets.

Wherever pain in erection, or heat of urine, or feverish symptoms, grow to any height, bleeding is the sovereign remedy. In reality, it should be used in all plethoric habits, and in every case where the pain is occasioned by excessive acrimony.

A truſs for the ſcrotum ſerves, beyond any thing, to keep off inflammation in the ſpermatic organs. It ſhould be worn from the firſt appearance of the diſeaſe, till it has ceaſed ſome weeks.

From what has been ſaid in deſcribing the different ſpecies of the gonorrhœa, it will eaſily be diſcovered, where the antiphlogiſtic plan is ſucceeding, where external applications will be uſeful, and likewiſe in what caſes recourſe muſt be had to the great ſpecific.

It has been generally believed, that the cure of the clap is beſt promoted by whatever encourages the diſcharge, particularly by briſk purgatives repeated daily, or at leaſt frequently. If by ſuch are meant reſins of jalap, and ſcammony, pulp of colocynth, and gamboge, I muſt diſapprove of their uſe, even though recommended by a Turner, a Sydenham, or a Boerhaave, who believed that the putrid
in-

infection was carried off by them moſt effectually. It ſeems to me, that they can only be warrantable, if given once or twice a week, and this in robuſt conſtitutions; ſince they always heat the body more or leſs, hurt the ſtomach, inflame the blood, and often bring on a ſtrangury or dyſury in a great degree, ſo as to increaſe the diſeaſe by every new doſe; or at beſt they produce the moſt tedious gleets.

When writers talk of fuſing the humours by ſuch purgatives, I would aſk what they mean. Are the humours fuſed, when fever is brought on, with great inflammation, ſwelled teſticles, and ſizy blood? Are the humours fuſed, where the running is ſtopt, and the virulence conveyed into the courſe of circulation, ſo as to occaſion ſpurious buboes, and glandular or lymphatic ſwellings, that are ſcarcely to be reſolved by flannel, mercury, ſarſa, or hemlock?

SECTION V.

Remarks on the first and second species.

WHAT has been now offered may be considered as containing general rules for the cure of the gonorrhœa. It may not be amiss to subjoin some particular observations, with respect to the first and second species, as before described, and distinguished; since they belong most properly to this stage of the distemper, and do not put on the pocky appearances which are often assumed by the rest, and which require on that account a very different management.

In the first, or most simple species of the gonorrhœa, a few doses of salts and manna dissolved in whey, and taken at the interval of two or three days, with quiet and sober living, will in the space of two

or

or three weeks produce a perfect cure. If matters muſt be hurried, injections may perhaps be uſed in the firſt ſpecies without much hazard; there being hardly morbid matter in ſuch quantity as to break in upon the habit. In this caſe, and in this alone, would I preſume to affirm, that mercury can never be neceſſary.

In the ſecond ſpecies, where ſo conſiderable a part of the diſeaſe is external, fomentations of the emollient kind, and poultices of wheat-bread and milk, frequently renewed, are of ſenſible benefit, if uſed along with the purgatives, &c. before preſcribed, unleſs where the infection is caught from a pocky patient, as happens frequently; in which caſe, the great ſpecific becomes abſolutely neceſſary.

SECTION VI.

General remarks.

IN every species of the clap, where there is inflammation, fomentations and poultices are useful, so far as they abate the heat and tension, preserve cleanliness, or promote the discharge.

When the cure is no longer dependent on the antiphlogistic method, Dr. Boerhaave seems to rest too much on their operation.

Milk and water of a proper warmth, in a half-pint stone vessel, in which the penis can be soaked twice or thrice a day, is sufficient for the general purpose of fomentation.

I said before, that any plan of medicine, or any regimen, exclusive of mercury, will not effect what I plead for, the curing speedily the virulent gonorrhœa,

rhœa, where it has been of long standing, or has got far back into the urethra. Inſtead therefore of expoſing the patient, by a ſevere and tedious purging courſe, to the hazard of a fever, and its attendants, viz. a checked diſcharge, and ſwelled teſticles, or perhaps a confirmed pox; I would propoſe that, as ſoon as there is a remiſſion in the heat of water and cordee, the inguina, pudenda, or thighs, ſhould be anointed with mercurial ointment as deſcribed below, or the blue or Belloſte's pill given twice a week, confiſting of ten grains to a doſe, and intermixed with the purging courſe at proper intervals. The conſequence of this treatment will be a ſpeedy amendment of the colour, and abatement of the diſcharge, as well as of all the ſymptoms, till they totally ceaſe.

By a judicious combination of the above methods, it is propoſed to remedy effectually

tually all the difficulties common in the fourth, fifth, and sixth species of the gonorrhœa.

SECTION VII.

*Of the swelled testicle.**

THE swelled testicle I mentioned in the first section as a circumstance peculiarly disagreeable. I have already observed, that it is generally produced by

---

* Having, in the year 1767, been to visit Mr. Heaviside at Hatfield, towards the autumn, I learned that there was an endemic disease in Hertfordshire, attended with a great and very painful swelling in the testes, and other symptoms as mentioned below.

Within a week of that time, a nobleman and two of his servants came up to London from the neighbourhood of Hatfield, and were seised with the mumps, &c. and not a little surprised at my prophesying, that in two or three days they would be seised with a swelling in the testes: it turned out just as I had foretold, and they recovered by a common antiphlogistic regimen. As I have never met with such a disease in my practice, nor ever read of any such, I take this op-

by daily and repeated draſtic purging, by being expoſed to cold during the courſe, or by living too freely, and taking too much exerciſe in the firſt ſtage of the diſeaſe, or by deſtructive injections. When I hint at the inflammation brought on in ſuch caſes, I would be underſtood to comprehend not only that affecting the teſticle itſelf, but its appendages, the epididymis, ſpermatic cord,
vaſa

opportunity of giving an account of it in the words of a letter from my very ingenious friend Mr. Hea‑viſide.

" IN the year 1767 I had a great many patients,
" the much greater part of them about or little paſt
" the age of puberty, ſeiſed with a diſorder very much
" reſembling what is called the Mumps, viz. with
" great ſtiffneſs and a conſiderable ſwelling about the
" articulation of the jaws. Some few complained a
" little, and but a little, of ſoreneſs in the throat;
" and a few had a faint raſh, chiefly about the neck
" and throat; both of which ſoon went off. They all
" of them had ſome degree of fever, attended with
" pain in the back. All theſe complaints, except the
" laſt, generally diſappeared about the third or fourth
" day, when there was a ſudden tranſlation of the
" matter

vasa deferentia, &c. which, without the strictest attention, end in sarcocele, suppuration, hydrocele, scirrhus, and cancer.

In the inflammatory stage, every one is agreed as to the propriety of bleedings, repeated according to circumstances, and likewise as to the utility of fomentations, with an antiphlogistic regimen of the severest

> matter to the testes, the fauces being immediately relieved and set at liberty. The inflammation and tension on the testes was very considerable in all of them, and in every respect resembling the hernia humoralis; but was quickly removed by gentle purges, cooling medicines, poultices to the part, and keeping quiet.—I remember I had two young girls, of about twelve or thirteen years old, seised with this complaint, where the humour was deposited on the labia pudendi. In none of the patients I saw (who were many) there was, or could be, the least suspicion of any venereal taint. I might add, that this distemper appeared again the next year, but more rarely; since when, or before, I never met with it."

Signed J. HEAVISIDE.

Hatfield, Hertfordshire,
April 11, 1772.

verest sort; that is, abstinence from meat, and even broths, as well as from all fermented liquors, excepting small beer. Where there is sizy blood, this is still absolutely necessary.

Dr. Sydenham, and many of our best surgeons, talk much of poultices of bean flower, litharge with vinegar, and many other detestable because so often pernicious preparations of this most deadly of all metals. But these render the solution of the inflamed part more difficult; and, what is much worse, produce such a scirrhus in the testicle, or its appendages, as is not to be resolved.

Poultices of bread and milk, with linseed flower, white lily roots, fenugreek seed, &c. are better calculated to promote the solution of the disease, by a discharge from the urethra of the obstructing, and perhaps virulent, matter. This is much the readiest way of clearing the testicle
per-

perfectly, without which there frequently remains an unconquerable gleet. So long therefore as any hardness continues in the testicle, or in the spermatic vessels, especially in the vas deferens, so long the testicle must be considered as a diseased body, and consequently subject to relapses, unless the habit be perfectly corrected by a proper antivenereal course.

The generality of writers have been extremely deficient in not marking, with sufficient accuracy, the mischiefs arising from the least neglect in this particular.

If at any time I find it impracticable to clear the testicle, by the antiphlogistic regimen now pointed out, and extended according to circumstances, I am never satisfied, till I have led the patient through such an antivenereal course, as shall ensure him against any future uneasiness from that quarter.

Besides

Besides rubbing mercury on the part (if free from pain) or on the inguina and thighs, I keep the testicle always suspended with a bag truss, and confine the patient to bed, for five or six weeks if necessary, fomenting the part with hemlock, and plying him inwardly with strong decoctions of sarsa, bardana, and extract of hemlock; not forgetting, all the while, to carry the mercurial unctions to their full extent.

I cannot forbear taking notice here of the singular use I have found in hemlock outwardly applied, as well as inwardly given; particularly in the case of B———, whose testicles had been both condemned to the knife. A scirrhosity, accompanying the hydrocele in each, and left by the operation, did still remain, notwithstanding a proper mercurial course, and an ample discharge by the digestion, till dissolved by hemlock.

By such methods I have cured diseased testicles of two or three years standing, even when ulcerated, and where the scirrhus had begun to be affected with pricking and lancing pains.

It is observable, that swellings of long continuance, which occasion the vasa deferentia to be knotted like a string of beads, are of very difficult resolution. Such a state requires a supine posture for the tedious space of six weeks, or perhaps more,* as well as a purulent or gleety discharge

* We have relieved a foreigner of rank from such a state of cancerous scirrhus, by obliging him, while under a severe regimen of diet, mercurial inunctions, fomentations, and strong decoctions of sarsaparilla, to lie above twenty hours in the four and twenty, for seven weeks, on his back, with his scrotum suspended, and his heels higher than his head. Castration had been recommended to this nobleman, by a person of distinguished reputation for dexterity and skill in the treatment of the venereal disease; but by the above regimen, the testicle, though of an enormous size, with hydrocele and lancing pains, was restored to a perfectly healthful

charge from the urethra, procured by means of bougies, aut fi a benevolo medico præferri liceat, gonorrhœâ recente, besides the resources above named.

Surely then, where copious discharges from the urethra prove so useful, the interrupting them by drying medicines, astringent applications, and injections, cannot fail in many cases to produce irremediable evils.

SECTION VIII.

Of gleets.

THIS is a word in every one's mouth, and made use of by many to cloak their ignorance with regard to the real cause which so often renders the disease obstinate,

ful state, and the water in the tunica propria testis was absorbed; in which happy situation he remains to this day.

ſtinate, as well as with relation to the proper method of removing it.

When the running continues beyond three weeks or a month, whether ſtill diſcoloured, or become clear and ropy, it is called a Gleet, and muſt be attacked with agglutinants, balſamics, and aſtringents, in every ſhape.

If the diſeaſe is ripe for ſuch medicines, it will ſtop by the uſe of ſome one or other of the claſs juſt mentioned,* or

---

* The beſt balſamic I know, where the ſtomach will bear ſo harſh a medicine, is the following:

℞. Gum. arabic. drach i.
    Balſam. copaiv.
    Mellis anglic. ana ſemi-unc. Simul conterentur, dein admiſce.
    Decoct. (fortior.) corticis peruv. unc. vii.
    Succ. limon. unc. i. Cujus mixtur. ſumat quartam partem m. & h. ſ. quotidie.

And the beſt aſtringent,

    A ſmall table ſpoonful of the tinct. ſtypt. (Ph. Londin.) out of a quarter of a pint of new milk, twice a day.

or even by abstaining totally from purging.

If, on the contrary, the matter is not ropy, but continues short like melted tallow, and the infection is still lurking in the part; such medicines will indeed often put a stop to the gleet, as it is called, and produce a confirmed pox. Almost every one knows this to be a fact; but how to prevent the bad effects of such a process, is known only to few.

It frequently happens, that the discharge continues for many months, in spite of every attempt by medicines given inwardly, as well as by injections. This is the great difficulty, and requires a more particular attention, as it is so common an evil.

To crush it in the bud, I would advise every young surgeon, at his first visits, to inform himself exactly as to the time when the running first began, and whether

ther it was attended with symptoms of cordee, heat of water, &c. or whether it is supposed to have risen from any former infection reappearing upon exercise, freer living, &c. and if so, to learn every circumstance of that infection, of its duration, and former treatment. He should likewise see the stream in which the urine flows, whether large, small, or scattered, in order to be acquainted with the exact state of the passage; for he may be sure, that old complaints there, lengthened out by the nature of the infection, by the particular habit of body, or by unskilful management, must have more or less affected the urethra, by contracting its diameter, or filling it with caruncles, which are very sensible to the touch of the bougie, though seldom seen upon dissection, at least as anatomists affirm.

If the discharge has manifestly the appearance of a fresh clap, attended with inflammatory

flammatory symptoms, it will be time enough to examine the urethra with a bougie, when, although your method of cure may have removed the inflammation, it has yet not carried off the gleet. In that case, it will help to save your own credit, as well as prevent much anxiety to your patient, if you examine whether its obstinacy be occasioned by any local complaint in the urethra. If the bougie passes freely, you will do well to set about the cure by a proper quantity of mercury rubbed on.

This quantity can, I think, be ascertained only by the change brought upon the matter, in respect of its colour or consistence. The surest signs, I know, of a tendency in the gleet to be dried up with speed and safety, are the appearances of little threads of matter, resembling vermicelli, floating in the urine as soon as made, or the stains on the linen becoming of small extent, not bigger than a pea.

Where

Where such change does not take place, as will sometimes happen, I rub on three or four ounces, so as scarcely to leave the possibility of a pocky cause remaining.

How many obstinate gleets of two, three, or four years standing, (and lately of seven and ten, in two foreigners of the first distinction) have we seen effectually cured by a mercurial inunction, when almost every other medicine had been tried in vain! Were we disposed to speculate, we should say, that in these cases an internal chancre had kept up the discharge, and that the discharge had preserved the body in such a state, as not to be greatly hurt by the continuance of the distemper.

Should the seat of the disease, or of the ulcer, lie about the prostate gland, callosities will be felt pretty distinctly near the anus, on the raphé or the perinæum, and generally attended with a strangury.

strangury. To determine with precision the place where these ulcers or chancres are formed, I know not any such proper method, next to that of using a bougie or a probe bent like a catheter, as desiring the patient, while he is making water, to press all along the urinary canal with his finger, till he comes to that point where the water in passing occasions most pain; for there probably the carnosities, scars, or strictures, are formed. To this point (after a thorough course of unction on the thighs) direct frictions, gummous, and resinous, or emollient applications outwardly, and bougies inwardly used with judgment and perseverance.

By these means, the passage will in most cases be again cleared, at least to a tolerable degree; the habit will be rectified, and the gleet dried up.

SECTION IX.

Of bougies.

ABOUT the middle of the sixteenth century, the nature of obstructions in the urethra began to be understood and treated with success by both regulars and empirics. Of the ingredients whereof bougies were composed we have several formulas in the books of that age, and their utility has been proved in every succeeding period.

Some years ago it was supposed, that an eminent writer on the maladies of the urethra possessed a composition of greater efficacy than any used by other surgeons; and his extraordinary success has been ascribed by the public to the peculiar properties of his bougies. Almost all the present writers contend, that the common bougie is as good as Mr. Daran's. But I must

I muſt needs ſay, that his method of applying them ſeems much better adapted to the nature of the complaint, than any other generally known. Who in this country, for example, perſeveres in their uſe with ſuch aſſiduity as that gentleman; beſides the ſlight of hand in introducing them, which he has acquired from having made it the ſtudy of his life? What ſurgeon but himſelf paſſes them twice or thrice a day, confines his patients to their couch, viſits them at a ſtated hour, regulates every meal and every cup of drink, increaſes and diminiſhes the ſize of the bougie,* changes the application according

---

* It ſeldom happens that the obſtruction in the urethra is of any great extent, but there are often three or four in the courſe of the paſſage. In either caſe, the very ſmall bougie is of no efficacy.

To paſs them readily, much depends on the point of the bougie being of the ſhape of a probe, or of a wedge. I have known two or three caſes, of many years

ing to circumstances, fixes their operation on the diseased part so nicely, or, by such extensive acquaintance with the principal difficulties of this kind throughout Europe, knows how to remedy them? In short, I cannot help thinking, that Mr. Daran is entitled to superior success by superior merit; at the same time that I acknowledge, he gives the whole a mysterious air, which favours more of quackery than of sound theory, or enlightened practice.

I have years standing, in which, by an attention to this circumstance, I have readily slipt the bougie through the obstruction, after fruitless attempts made by others, to the infinite relief and comfort of the patients; and very lately in three elderly men, who had been tortured, as they supposed, with the stone and gravel, for which they had taken lithontriptics of every kind, for years together. I have found, on examination of the urinary passage by a bougie, that an obstruction in the urethra, from a venereal injury fifteen or twenty years before, was the source of all their misery; and to which neither they, nor their physicians, had attended. They are now restored to health and joy.

I have not been able to discover why Dr. Astruc prefers the leaden bougies to the common sort, or why he represents the last, of which we all know so much good, as ineffectual.

I cannot leave the article of bougies, without mentioning a case I lately met with, of a kind of impotence arising from a stricture very near the glans penis; where it occurred to me, that an obstruction so near the point might, on attempting coition, affect the seminal vesicles so sensibly as always to occasion the semen being thrown off, ante vestibulum orci: and so it was in fact; for, by the use of the bougies, the obstruction was speedily removed. I was told by my patient's wife, that I had been of great service, and that, if her husband had applied to me sooner, he might have been cured long ago. The good woman lies in at this time.

SECTION X.

Of buboes.

MUCH has been written about venereal buboes, enough to confound even those who are not beginners. The following facts concerning them are true, and may I hope be useful to explain the difficulties that occur on this part of the subject.

Buboes appear singly, as well as accompanied with other venereal symptoms. Before they come to maturity, the patient is generally oppressed about the præcordia; which does not, I think, happen in any degree of comparison, under any other circumstance of the pox. As soon as the matter flows off, the patient is greatly relieved, though they do not heal without a relapse, (even where they have not appeared, till after the venereal course has

has been thought complete) unless indeed they are assisted by persevering in that course, or by mercurial alteratives.

The French practice of repelling buboes, and purging them off, I have not found to answer, though tried with the utmost care. Rubbing the mercurial ointment on the bubo itself, serves only to repel the disease into the habit, let the quantity rubbed on be ever so proper. Ulcers in the throat, or foul bones, are often the immediate consequence. And here, once for all, I declare loudly against every mercurial application to the diseased or ulcerated part, in every venereal case; till the general habit is thoroughly rectified by a proper course.

Perhaps indeed there is one exception to this rule, viz. where, in a fresh clap, the patient is threatened with a phymosis during the inflammatory stage of the distemper; when the ointment, rubbed on the

the prepuce and glans penis, preserves the part from ulcerations, until the running and regimen have given the disease a milder form.

If the bubo is not from its first appearance attended with considerable pain, its suppuration will advance slowly; and therefore the patient should not wait for it, but immediately set about his cure with mercurial ointment, and suffer the bubo to take its chance, yet using the utmost caution not to let the ointment get near the bubo itself; otherwise he may increase his disease by a digestive regimen, and give it time to spread by delaying the use of the specific. The whole should be allowed to ripen, before it is opened. Provided the blood be otherwise in a good state, it will soon heal, and fill up, even if opened only by a longitudinal incision, without torturing the edges with the knife, or destroying them by caustic applications.

If

If the blood and juices be tainted with a scorbutic, scrophulous, or cancerous quality,* the sore will not soon look kindly, whether treated in the way of any outward application, or of any internal course. In the scorbutic and scrophulous state, antiscorbutics, strengtheners, and open air, will mend the appearances, and heal the sores, if a sufficient quantity of mercury has been likewise used. It is in the case of scrophula chiefly, that mercury does most mischief, notwithstanding what the celebrated Ballonius says of its virtues in the struma.

I have never met with any incurable cancerous buboes. They have indeed often gone on for many months; but they have always disappeared, as the habit mended.

* I have often lamented that there was not a law prohibiting marriage among scrophulous, maniac, and cancerous constitutions, as well as against wedlock before puberty.

mended.* Of late years at leaſt, opium given inwardly, and preparations of hemlock both outwardly and inwardly adminiſtered, have, with the aſſiſtance of country air and a heartier diet, hardly ever failed to promote a digeſtion, and effect a cure in a reaſonable time. To ſay the truth, I have, in many caſes where I could give no relief by other means, experienced ſuch frequent good effects of Storck's hemlock, and aconite medicines, as convince me, that there has been ſome want of candour in crying them down ſo ſtrongly without fairer trials. I have, for ſome years paſt, given above ten pound weight of the extract of cicuta annually, in which time, it is certain

* When buboes have not been well managed, or are opened by art, or break before the venereal hardneſs is melted down into pus, they become ſpurious. In ſuch caſes, mercury in any ſhape, or even applied to the part, will not diſſolve the hardneſs; but I have ſeen them give way in a few days to decoction of ſarſaparilla, a quart a day.

I have both frequently succeeded, and frequently failed. I have failed however seldomer in mending the face of cacoëthic sores, than in any other circumstance.

SECTION XI.

Of chancres.

WHERE there is not venereal virus sufficient to produce any other symptom but a chancre on the præputium, or glans penis, I consider the case as the most simple species of pox, but yet hardly ever, perhaps I should say never, to be cured radically, without a mercurial course. A plentiful discharge from the chancre, promoted by emollient and detergent-applications, if not of the mercurial kind, will, no doubt, forward the cure considerably: but I am forced to differ from Dr. Boerhaave and others, when they suppose the appearance in question to be a local complaint only, and such as may be cured by external applications. Let it be added, that every mercurial application to the chancre itself, whether in the shape of ointment, or of mercury in solutis principiis, as the chemists affect to call it, will for the most part only hide the disease, or drive it to the inguinal and axillary glands, to the tonsils, or even to the bones themselves, unless a complete antivenereal course be pursued; and yet nothing is more common than dressing the chancre with every species of mercurial dressings. Nor is any practice more usual than the putting such a patient on a course of purgatives with mercurials intermixed; which method often produces a running from the urethra, and translates the chancre to its internal surface. No sooner is this effected, than it passes for a gleet only, and

the

the chancre is forgot; turpentines and other balsamics are prescribed, the running stops, and the surgeon, who acts on such a plan, takes his leave. Observe the consequence: On the first debauch, or violent exercise, the gleet returns; and if the unhappy patient has been again living at large, the running is considered as a fresh infection; at best he is put on a purging course for twenty or thirty days, without any change on the colour of the discharge, or diminution in its quantity; and after six weeks it is referred to a former taint, and the same cruel game is played with the constitution, which without the strength of a Hercules, the patience of a Job, and the assistance of a master in the profession, ends in an incurable gleet, or leaves the urethra in a chancrous state, full of strictures and carnosities..

SECTION XII.

Of other pocky symptoms.

AFTER what has been already said on the nature of venereal infection, and the method of treating it in the circumstances above stated, it will generally be understood how to apply the doctrine to all the other appearances of the disease, however multiplied. But let it be still remembered, that the more numerous the marks of infection are, the more necessary it will be to attend to the quality of the constitution, to the quantity of mercury requisite, and the regimen adapted to both.

It will naturally be asked here, Does the whole cure then consist in using a proper quantity of mercurial ointment, with a proper attention to those few circumstances? I answer, that, where

the

the body is otherwife in perfect health, it generally does; not elfe. For example, a man catches the difeafe after a long fea voyage, or a fevere campaign: in this cafe, though perhaps to outward appearance all looks well, the blood is yet often fo much diftempered, that the fymptoms foon grow untoward, or fhow themfelves obftinate, and the patient is broke down, before you are aware. Or fuppofe he has got a clap only; the heat of urine continues beyond the ufual period, the erections are frequently intolerable, the cordee remains for weeks together, erofions behind the glans penis make their appearance, and this fo equivocal that you can fcarce fay to what degree the infection is advanced, and neither purging nor mercurials are effectual, fo as greatly to perplex the patient, and perhaps not a little to puzzle the phyfician.

If it happens to be the pox, and the chancres cannot be brought to a kindly difcharge, but on the contrary fpread and inflame, the bubo will neither fuppurate, nor can it be healed; and if the difeafe by neglect, or by the malignity of the infection, becomes more complicated, and lefs governable, the ufual treatment fails. The fame thing takes place, to a greater or lefs degree, in a fcrophulous or cancerous habit, and produces almoft infuperable difficulties, unlefs the patient is fortunate enough to fall into the hands of a man of medical learning, or large experience, who knows how to reftore the blood to a balfamic ftate, and thereby to difentangle the infection from the habit with efficacy, certainty, and fpeed.

To promote fuch a ftate of the juices, was probably the caufe of introducing the ufe of diet drinks, almoft as foon as this malady was known; and in countries
where

where the perspiration is excessive, and the fluids are thin, the contagion was to be carried off by the balsamic or active qualities of those drinks.

It will, I am afraid, be reckoned a kind of heresy to maintain, that the guaiacum is of little or no virtue in the venereal disease. Volumes have been written to extol its powers. Dr. Boerhaave has rendered the name of Hutten immortal, by the manner in which he espouses his method of giving it. True it is, he wrote in Holland, and, it may be generally presumed, with a peculiar eye to Dutch constitutions, or phlegmatic habits, in which this medicine might possibly succeed. Thus much however I can freely affirm, that I have given it, or seen it given, times without number, in almost all the stubborn symptoms of the disorder under consideration, without the least efficacy, unless in habits that were

very

very phlegmatic indeed, or elſe greatly impoveriſhed, or laſtly where it has been combined with the ſarſaparilla.

To what I have advanced elſewhere concerning the virtues of ſarſaparilla I would only add here, that I have not ſince the year 1753, when I firſt gave it in ſtrong decoctions, found any reaſon to retract the leaſt part of what I then aſſerted; excepting only in the caſe of a few cancerous buboes, which will not, I believe, give way on a ſudden to any method hitherto diſcovered,* but which, I know,

may

---

* Since the above was written, M'Donald, a centinel in the third regiment of foot-guards, had a truly cancerous bubo, that extended above a foot in diameter on the abdominal muſcles, for which every thing was tried in vain, where the diſcharge and pain had reduced the patient almoſt to a ſkeleton. It occurred to me, that lemon juice might poſſibly be uſeful: I ordered him half a dozen of lemons, or upwards, in a day, which he devoured with the ſame eagerneſs as if they had been apples. He had not done this for three days together, when all his pains ceaſed, the ſores yielded

may be gradually subdued, either by fresh air, fuller diet, abstinence from mercurials, or by hemlock applied outwardly, or given inwardly, whether with or without opiates. My assertion in the Medical Essays of London, vol. 1st,* was, 'That 'every case truly venereal is manageable 'by mercury, or by sarsa combined with 'mercury.'

As yielded the whitest and mildest matter, and contracted beyond belief, so as to heal in two or three weeks. Since that time I have never seen any difficulty in healing the most obstinate bubo, where there was pain, ragged edges, or cancerous appearances, provided a proper quantity of mercury had been previously applied; nor any inconvenience from mercurial medicines, where (I will call it) the scorbutic habit had been rectified by the lemon-juice. My experienced and judicious friend Mr. Wollaston, surgeon to the third regiment of foot-guards, has ever since, both in private and public, practised this method with success. The necessity of this note will appear from some important observations on the subject, in the second volume of the Medical Transactions of London, page 338 et infra.

* See the Appendix.

As to decoctions of bardana and mezereon roots, the herbs saponaria, lobelia, &c. which have been cried up by different writers, my experience of their powers has been too small to enable me to pronounce with certainty, but quite sufficient to incline me to speak doubtfully, concerning them.

SECTION XIII.

Necessary remarks on the disease.

THE venereal disease differs from most others in this respect, that it has no perfect crisis, except in its simplest species.

It is always in a progressive state, growing worse every hour, and recoiling with double force, if the cure be interrupted by irregularity of any kind, or if you give over the antivenereal regimen before the complaint is fairly conquered.

It

It differs in its quality from itself, as much as the confluent small pox differs from the most distinct sort.

In its most inflammatory state, the antidote may be applied so injudiciously as to throw it much deeper into the habit, than it would advance in equal time, if left to the treatment usual in other inflammatory diseases.

The constitution is able to throw off a considerable portion of the infectious matter by the urethra in a gonorrhœa, and by the suppuration of a bubo in a confirmed pox, with much more ease than by purging in the clap, or by a mercurial course singly in the pox. In the last however, as we hinted before, such a discharge alone we have never found sufficient, though we have repeatedly made the experiment.

It falls out but rarely, that the disease in our days affects the viscera with such

such obstructions as it produced at its first appearance, when the gonorrhœa had not yet shewed itself, and the use of mercury was less understood. This indeed I have met with in three or four cases, where the antivenereal plan only had power to remove the evil.

I am informed that the Asiatics cure many dropsies, and obstructed viscera, by anointing the hepatic region with mercurial ointment. The obstructions so cured have been probably owing to a venereal cause. I have failed in two or three instances where the trial was made very faithfully, but where I had no reason to believe that there was any thing venereal in the habit.

Antiscorbutic and tonic medicines, oranges, lemons, and vegetables, particularly the hemlock and bark, must pave the way to the cure of this disorder, if you wish that cure to be expeditious and lasting,

lasting, in the case of scorbutic or scrophulous constitutions, where venereal complaints are always peculiarly dangerous.

It is a declaration due to truth, that I have not, in any preparation of mercury used by injection, found either a certain preventive, or a certain cure, of any venereal taint, at any season from or before coition to the most complete virulent gonorrhœa, notwithstanding the boasted powers of nostrums which Fallopius, Musitanus, F. Hoffman, and many profound connoisseurs, and I will add, unprincipled impostors in this metropolis, so confidently recommend.

Certain it is that I have formerly brought a pox on several, by attempting a cure with injections of calomel, mercurial ointment dissolved with the yolk of an egg and injected, mercurial ointment introduced into the urethra, the famed solution of mercury with gum ammoniac,

diluted

diluted aqua phagædenica, and Van Swieten's aqua antivenerea, &c.*

Musitanus indeed goes so far as to affirm, that he has known a thousand claps cured by an injection of calomel. We have seen many obstinate gleets cured by it, at the end of a proper course; but must repeat, that we have brought the pox on several people in the clap, by means of this medicine, when we used it in the beginning of a gonorrhœa virulenta.

F. Hoffman has asserted the same thing with the priest; but neither of their authorities can weigh against daily observation.

---

* Notwithstanding the bold asseverations of our modern injection-mongers, I am convinced, by every new day's experience, of the many mischiefs arising from stopping runnings in recent claps by injections. A man of honour and veracity has within these few days assured me, that fifty of his acquaintances, besides himself, have been poxed lately by the injections of one surgeon in this town.

SECTION XIV.

A problem.

WHAT pains have not been taken to find out an application, or injection, that will, either ante aut post coïtum, prevent venereal infection? Fallopius, Musitanus, and others, have given us prescriptions, of whose efficacy they seem to entertain no doubt.

To me, I confess, the subtilty of this poison appears too like that of electrical fire to be prevented. It is well for the human race that it can be cured.

I knew a young man, whose blood was obliged to be loaded with mercury in a great quantity by inunction for a pocky taint. As soon as his cure was completed, he lay with a woman who infected every body else, but he escaped. In this case, I suppose, the quantity of mercury in the habit overbalanced the quantity of disease, and acted as a prophylactic: 'mais le jeu ne vaut pas la chandelle.'

'Forsan hydrargyrum in oleo animali vel vegetabili cocto solutum, et virgæ ante coïtum benè inunctum, ad prophylaxin appropinquat.'

SECTION XV.

Of mercury and its preparations.

SOON after the venereal distemper had made its appearance in our hemisphere, it was discovered, that medicines of the common sort neither checked ts progress, nor accomplished its cure. Some of the symptoms resembling so nearly those obstinate diseases where mercurial medicines alone had been found effectual, probably led our forefathers to try their efficacy in this, notwithstanding its supposed bad qualities, which they attempted to correct by the addition of other ingredients. The malignity and spread of the difeafe foon brought it into general ufe.

Who has not heard of the changeable nature of mercury from a fluid into a folid, from a volatile into a fixed ftate, from a mild into an acrid quality, and from its own colour into almoft all colours? The chemifts, or the alchemifts, can tell you how all this happens, and lover-like are fondeft of what has given them moft trouble. To them I refer the curious enquirer, meaning only to lay before my reader a few facts concerning mercury, and its preparations, that may claim fome attention from thofe who have the care of venereal cafes.

And firft, as to its ores; the virtues of thefe do not by any means correfpond with what has been faid of them in moft books that treat of venereal difeafes.

M 2   For

For native cinnabars are, in their effects on the body, either fettered on the one hand by their combination with sulphur, or dangerous on the other by effluvia from the arsenical part of them. I have twice seen a considerable salivation raised by giving native cinnabar inwardly. The mischiefs occasioned by fumigations, where the lungs are weak, or subject to asthmas, hæmorrhages, &c. are well known. The disappointments I have met with from the use of the factitious, or antimonial kinds, both given inwardly, and outwardly applied, correspond exactly with the experience of Dr. Astruc on this head. But I feel very little disposition to try powers which are at best equivocal, where we have certain ones at hand. I mean, that their application represses, or at best only translates the complaints for which they are used, rather than extirpates them.

If quickfilver, when strained through leather,

leather, leaves no dregs behind, or diſtilled with quick-lime comes out in the ſame quantity as when put into the veſſel, it is then fit for every uſe, whether outwardly applied or inwardly adminiſtered, as well as for all the preparations into which chemiſts have tortured it.

In the courſe of experiments recorded by Engliſh writers, it appears, that large quantities of quickſilver, even to the amount of ſixteen pound weight,* have been

---

* Having accidentally heard my friend William Fiſher, Eſq. of Camberwell, in Surry, mention two caſes, and confiſtent with his knowledge, very extraordinary both for the quantity of crude mercury taken inwardly, and its effects; I have added a copy of a letter which he has favoured me with on this ſubject.

"*Camberwell, April* 11, 1772.
" DEAR SIR,
" IN conſequence of your requeſt, I ſend you
" an account of two gentlemen of my acquaintance,
" who each of them told me they had taken above
" one hundred pounds weight of crude mercury
" W.

been swallowed by one patient, without producing any remarkable phænomena in

"W. Moses, whose letter is published page 158, in Dr. Dover's Legacy, is one of them: and he told me he never walked one mile without sitting down, before he took quicksilver; and that, after taking three hundred and sixty-five ounces in so many days, he walked to Batson's coffee-house from Greenwich, to tell Dr. Dover how well he was, and after drinking a dish of chocolate he walked back again; and that he has had a quantity come from him after he had not taken any for six months. The above was a lieutenant in the navy, and then about forty-six years old when he told me the tale, and something short-breathed: he thought he could not have lived, if he had not taken the above.

"The other was a gentleman of Putney, extremely afflicted with the rheumatism, laid up almost all winter for years; and when he told me, which was in April, (thirty-five years since) he said his practice was, last winter, to shoot; and when wet to the skin, he went to the club after he came home, and found no hurt from sittting till his clothes dried on his back.

"I sincerely believe both accounts to be true, and am,

"Dear Sir,
"Yours, &c.
"W. FISHER."

in that cafe, or indeed in any other; unlefs when a part of it happened to be diffolved by the faliva, or gaftric juices, and thereby lodged for fome time in the primæ viæ, where it produced the common effect of increafing the falivary fecretions, in proportion to the quantity diffolved, or to the ftate of the patient's juices at the time of giving it. In thefe inftances it correfponds with mercury diffolved in honey, turpentine, &c. as in the pil. Barbaroff. de Belloft, pil. mercurial. Pharm. Lond. &c. at the worft producing fymptoms very manageable in general, and effects more or lefs beneficial according to circumftances.

As to the effects of crude mercury in this difeafe, diffolved with turpentines, or otherwife combined with alexipharmics, diuretics, purgatives, &c. I would not abfolutely fay, that the pocky infection is always too great for fuch medicines

to

to take place: but fo long as you remain ignorant in what proportion the mercurial medicine has entered the lacteal veffels, and what points it has carried, you cannot tell how to afcertain the dofe, or fecure the patient againft a relapfe; that is, in pocky cafes.

The fame objection, though not in the fame degree, lies againft trufting to its effect in plafters: for, on the firft appearance of the difeafe, much was done by them both in their fimple and complicated forms, provided they were perfevered in long enough to lodge a fufficient quantity.

He muft be a man of very little obfervation indeed, who has not feen the mifchiefs arifing from mercurial plafters applied to buboes, and other venereal tumours, by fending them back into the habit.

Let us now fee what is affected by ointment prepared in the moft fimple form,

or

or crude mercury rubbed into an ointment with an equal quantity of hogs-lard.

In the virulent gonorrhœa, mercurial ointment having been rubbed on the groins in juft proportions, fuppofe to the quantity of an ounce or more at due intervals (purgative medicines being intermixed at proper diftances); the difcharge generally changes from a green or yellow colour to one whiter, and more refembling the femen, or to one of a yellow tinge in the middle of the fpeck; or elfe it becomes more ropy, and lefs like melted tallow, diminifhing at the fame time in quantity. But where the gonorrhœa has been of fuch long ftanding as to have produced carnofities or ftrictures in the urethra, no inunction will be fufficient without a local treatment.

When the difeafe fhews itfelf with pocky fymptoms, as chancres, buboes, puftules, &c. and you rub on a due proportion of this ointment, accompanied with a suitable regimen, what are the effects? Sometimes a plentiful spitting, with its attendants, and a cure; sometimes plentiful sweating, and a cure; at other times no sensible evacuation, or change on the body, and yet a cure, equally agreeable and permanent; except in some few cases, which are conquered afterwards by diet drinks, small doses of pil. argent. vivi, or slight mercurial frictions.

I allow that the diminution of the symptoms is not always apparent, however properly the course may have been pursued, and that thirty or even forty drachms of the strong mercurial ointment will not always remove the symptoms of the disease. Continue, in that case, to rub a few times more, and a larger quantity at a time; and what ensues? As if the artillery had not been heavy enough before, by thus increasing its weight you make a breach

at

at laſt, and the diſeaſe is taken by ſtorm; frequently, as was ſaid above, without ſalivation, ſweating, a greater diureſis, or any diſagreeable conſequence whatever; and generally too without any ſeverity of regimen, even in open air. I would not be underſtood to mean, that the inunctions are, in this event, to be left off immediately. On the contrary, it ſhould be a general rule to continue them for a ſhorter or longer time, according to the degree of ſtubbornneſs which has attended the ſymptoms; as it is certain that, without ſuch precaution, there may be a danger of their returning.

The two oldeſt and moſt experienced ſurgeons in the treatment of venereal complaints, that I am acquainted with, have both aſſured me, that a very great part of the miſchief done by this diſeaſe in England, ſeemed to have ariſen from want of

at-

attention to the proper quantity of mercury neceffary for its abfolute extinction.

In relation to this quantity, hear the opinion of two celebrated judges among foreigners. "It is difficult," fays Aftruc,*
"to affert, à priori, what quantity of
"mercury will, in the whole, be necef-
"fary to cure the diftemper completely;
"fince that depends upon the age, fex,
"and temperament of the patient; the
"malignity, degree, and inveteracy of the
"infection; the number, ufe, and im-
"portance of the parts affected. It
"muft be judged of à pofteriori, from
"the abatement and ceafing of the
"fymptoms; but it is found by repeated
"obfervations, that commonly not lefs
"than two ounces of the ftrong mercu-
"rial ointment is fufficient, and not more
"than three or four ounces neceffary."

The

* Aftruc, lib. iv. cap. 7. p. 272. ed. Parif. 1740, 4to.

The other writer, Septalius, who had the care of the great hospital of Broglio at Milan, for forty years together, where by his account he cured of the venereal disease near one thousand patients yearly, says,* " That for completing one cure there ought to be used, at repeated inunctions, three or four ounces of quicksilver; and that the infection should not be carried off by purgatives, unless in cases of the utmost necessity." It is the advice of this experienced physician,† either not to use mercurials at all, or to use them in a quantity sufficient to ensure success; " since by too sparing an application of them the morbid matter is set in motion; and the symptoms being only diminished, not removed, unless perhaps to the nobler parts, the patient is left,

" un-

---

* Septalii Animad. lib. vii. § 224 & 231.
† Id. lib. vii. § 218.

"uncured and disappointed, to drag out a miserable life."

I question whether any omission in the practice of physic hurts so deeply the health of the rising generation, as that just now mentioned. Let me call upon the young and ingenuous practitioners of the healing art, as they value the honour of their profession, and the welfare of their fellow creatures, not to neglect this counsel from one who has been using mercury near thirty years, for almost as many venereal patients as Septalius himself.

I cannot restrain myself from observing here, how fashionable it is become with many to despise old writers, and to depreciate as obsolete every observation, how useful soever in practice, that has not been made in our more enlightened days: but, certainly, he who has established the truest principles of cure de-

serves

serves the greatest esteem, and the closest attention, at whatever period he wrote.

With regard to the composition of the ointment, I would always recommend equal proportions of lard and quicksilver; the inunction with a drachm or two, at most, being with difficulty rubbed on to dryness, without leaving the thighs too long exposed to the air; as on the other hand a quantity of mercury sufficient to extinguish the infection, is not easily rubbed on, if the proportion of lard to quicksilver be double.

When the patient's skin is easily fretted, the ointment should be prepared with as small a quantity of turpentine as possible; by which means he is saved an eruption of angry pustules, that often obstruct the anointing of those parts where it can be done most completely, namely the thighs, and the inside of them especially. When such pustules are troublesome, the
oint-

ointment must be applied on the outsides, till the insides of the thighs have recovered.

By the way, one is tempted to smile at the common manner of applying the mercurial ointment, first on the feet, then on the legs, then on the thighs, then on the arms, shoulders, and trunk of the body; as if there were magic in the process, and the doctor were a conjurer. Surely the ointment rubbed upon the thighs, which can be defended from cold in winter by flannel drawers, and in summer by cotton or linen ones, worn during the whole time of the inunction, and where it can be applied without any inconveniency, is as well or better calculated to convey the mercury into the blood, though not to keep up the parade of art.

Too large a quantity should not be made at once. The unguentum cœruleum

leum fortius, of the London Pharmacopiœa, should be expunged as ineffectual, in any confiderable degree, for the cure of the venereal difeafe; the balfam of fulphur, with which the mercury is combined, probably deftroying its efficacy; at leaft I have found it fo.

If any confiderable quantity of the ointment is prepared at once, it should be ftirred up from the bottom of the pot every time it is ufed, that the whole may be equally ftrong.

It is not an uncommon practice to anoint the joints with the mercury. I have heard people, who have been fo treated, complain of great coldnefs in them afterwards. Surely it is more probable that an abforption of the mercury on the tendinous or nervous parts of our frame should produce fuch fymptoms, fince, we are told that artificers, and the workers

ers of mercurial mines, are subject to them on the fleshy parts of the thighs.

I pretend not to decide whether the lard's becoming attenuated by age is an advantage or no. Septalius touches on these two last particulars.

The following hints deserve the notice of every surgeon, and are not generally known.

Rub a little, suppose less than a drachm at a time, of mercurial ointment upon a chancre, a beginning bubo, or phymosis, and repeat it daily for three or four times; and it will remove the appearance of disease from the part, and drive it into the constitution, perhaps upon the bones, probably into the throat, but always from the part. Every mercurial application to a venereal sore, whether chancre or bubo, is equally improper, till you have conquered the infection.

Rub to the quantity of three, four,

or

or five, and some few times more ounces, in proper doses, upon any part of the body, except the part affected; and all the symptoms of the disease, which deserve the name of venereal, will either disappear, and never return, or else be so altered as to give way to diet drinks of sarsa, or bardana, or perhaps of the plants saponaria and lobelia, or the roots of mezereon. Of the sarsaparilla I speak with certainty; of the others, the longer I live, I doubt the more.

Again, rub a small quantity of the mercurial ointment on any part of the body, in the case of a scrophulous or scorbutic habit, tainted at the same time with the pox; and, in many instances, it will produce a violent salivation, that in spite of all sorts of remedies shall run on for several weeks; the patient shall be much reduced in his strength, wasted in his body, and remain tainted with the discase, notwithstanding the salivation has been so inordinate. Repeat the anointing, and the effect will be the same, though in a less degree.

But first correct this scorbutic disposition, then rub on the mercury, proceed to the length above mentioned, at proper intervals, and in proper quantities; and you will generally, even without affecting the mouth, obtain a complete cure. Go beyond this quantity, and, except in a few cases, mercury shall seem to have produced no further effect on the symptoms. Here we may say with truth, that it has done both its best, and its worst: it has saved the constitution from being ruined by the disease, and it has changed a strong into a weaker habit.

Formerly, physicians were exceeding solicitous to raise the salivation to the utmost height, lest they should not be certain of the cure without it. Of late, they

they have been contented with sweating, or plentiful discharges of urine. Now, many are satisfied if they use a given quantity, whether it affects the salivary glands, or goes off either by perspiration or urine. I am disposed to be of the last number, with this difference, that where there is a little soreness and heat in the gums, I should expect a more speedy cure, than where there is either none at all, or where there is a more copious salivation.

I have sometimes gone so far as to think, that mercury, by producing a sort of fermentation in the juices, without loading too much the salivary glands, or augmenting their secretions considerably, was better for the constitution, than when, by greatly tainting the saliva, it produced a putrid diathesis. More experience has confirmed me in this idea.

Upon the whole, I believe, that purging gently in the inflammatory state, at the intervals already specified, and intermixing crude mercury internally, or applying it externally in just quantities, as soon as the symptoms of inflammation are abated, will cure a clap in all its stages; and that mercurial ointment, used in the proportions above directed, will generally secure the constitution against the further progress of a confirmed pox, or at least enable you to eradicate it by the assistance of other medicines before mentioned.

I hope that delicate patients will not be alarmed at such a method of cure, when I shall have mentioned one fact, viz. that, in the course of near thirty years practice, I have not been able to trace any lasting bad effects of mercury on those who have used even the largest quantities of it, by inunction, in the case of constitutions otherwise healthy. I speak not of scorbutic, scrophulous, cancerous, nor yet of paralytic ones, where family
infirmities

infirmities are moſt injuriouſly imputed to mercury.

Compare now the effects of mercurial ointment juſt deſcribed, with thoſe of mercury in ores, but chiefly diſſolved with acids; in which I include the turpeths, corroſive ſublimate, or the latter dulcified by repeated ſublimations, and mercurial precipitates. Of ſome of theſe a quarter or half a grain, or even leſs, and that diluted too, will produce anxieties, tremblings, vomitings, hypercatharſes, convulſions, and ſometimes death; at beſt, ſalivations not to be reſtrained for weeks, months, or even a longer period. I know, at this moment, an old patient of mine, who has returns of the ſalivation, that laſt for weeks together, accompanied with a braſſy taſte in his mouth, as if he was under a courſe of mercury, though it is now above twelve years ſince he has uſed any, in whatever ſhape. And, what is perhaps yet more to be dreaded, no cure, or not a permanent one, will be accomplished at last, though the salivation be repeated. Yet some or all of these dreadful consequences must be hazarded, because a smaller quantity of mercury in this way is pretended to be sufficient for the cure, and less destructive, as well as more delicate. The last part of the proposition I admit, but the other two I utterly deny.

Were it right to give into theory, on a subject where we have facts sufficient; it might perhaps be said of mercury acidulated in any way you will, that even the salivation, with all its severe attendants, is not your security. Either the sores do not heal, or the symptoms do not disappear, perhaps indeed from the patient's not being able to bear the severity of the salivation, and the repeated effects of the mercury on the stomach or bowels; or finally no cure takes place.

SEC-

SECTION XVI.

On the present state of the pox.

IT is a question that has been much agitated, whether the disease of which we have been treating, is on the decline or not. I would answer it by asking another question, Is the passion for pleasure on the decline?

In fact, I believe that the disease is growing much more general, while the treatment of it is still shamefully unequal.

There has been an æra in its history, when it became milder. I allude to the first appearance of the gonorrhœa. But too many surgeons daily shut up that avenue to relief, by a variety of injections mercurial, balsamic, and astringent. I leave their patients to bear witness with what woful effects; amongst others, swelled testicles, unhappy wives, and an half rotten posterity.

Another principal source of the increase of this evil is the general ignorance with regard to the quantity of mercury requisite, and to the manner of applying it, which changes totally the face and quality of the complaint.

A third most material circumstance to be reckoned here is that of the grafts from Africa, and both the Indies; where, the treatment being still less understood, the disease has been suffered to lay deeper hold, and to produce more stubborn symptoms.

The last cause that I shall mention, but not the least, is the constitution of modern livers; where love of ease, love of pleasure, continual watching, and anxious gaming, have miserably enervated the posterity of those heroes who fought at Agincourt and Cressy.

THE END.

APPENDIX.

ON THE VIRTUES OF THE SARSAPARILLA ROOT IN THE VENEREAL DISEASE.*

THE reputation that a certain medicine has of late years acquired in London in some venereal cases, and in which the sarsaparilla is supposed to be the principal ingredient, put me upon enquiring among my friends if any experiments had been made to verify such a conjecture.

* First published in the Medical Observations of London.

It was in the courfe of this enquiry that Dr. Hunter favoured me with the hiftory of a venereal cafe, attended with ill conditioned ulcers in the groin, wherein a ftrong decoction of the farfaparilla root, taken to the quantity of a quart a day, and perfifted in for fome time, had effected a cure; when a mercurial courfe and other things had failed.

For my own fatisfaction I refolved to profecute this hint, and make a trial of the farfaparilla root in a number of cafes, fo as to difcover if the fuccefs of the above-mentioned remedy in many cafes, particularly where almoft every other medicine had failed, was not chiefly owing to this ingredient.

Thefe experiments, with their good or bad fuccefs, I have been induced to offer to the public; the rather, as I cannot but flatter myfelf that I have now made a fufficient number of obfervations to enable me

to

to deduce some general rules for using the sarsaparilla with a probability of success, and at the same time ascertaining the virtues of a valuable medicine, hitherto much neglected, or little understood; though it has been always ranked among the efficacious medicines in the venereal disease, by most authors who have written on that subject.

CASE I.

About the month of August 1751, Mrs. Marshall, a carpenter's wife in Long-acre, applied to me for a complaint she had in her breast, where I found the nipple much corroded by a painful chancre, attended with many venereal blotches all round her breast. Upon examining her throat I found foul ulcers on both sides: I learned on enquiry, that she had contracted this disease by suckling for a few days a neighbour's

bour's child, whofe mouth and lips were full of venereal chancres; but fhe at that time had no fufpicion of its having any venereal fymptoms, or that fhe could be infected by it. Her having no previous mark of the difeafe, and her hufband, who cohabited with her all the time, enjoying perfect health, had prevented her hitherto from afking advice; and then fhe did it principally on her child's account, which fhe had fuckled, who was at that time about fix months old, and who had many blotches on its body, with large fici about its anus. Not doubting any longer of the way in which fhe had contracted the difeafe, fhe, by my advice, went to one of the hofpitals, where fhe was falivated, and after fix weeks was difmiffed apparently in good health; but in two months time fhe had a return of her fore throat, with the additional fymptoms of violent pains
all

all over her head. In February 1751-2, she applied to me again: as I found her throat well, and her breast had not the foul appearance as formerly, I hoped that the pains in her head might proceed from a different cause, and might give way to nervous medicines, which were ordered her, but without effect. The ulcers in her throat becoming foul again, I could no longer doubt of her being still poxed: I then used fumigations of cinnabar to her throat, gave her preparations of antimony, with the antiscorbutics, strong decoctions of guaiacum, and a small proportion of sassafras and sarsaparilla; by which means the throat grew tolerably well, but the head-ache continued: notwithstanding which she became pregnant in the summer 1752. Three months after, all her bad symptoms returned with more violence than ever, with pains about her palate and in her nose, and the ulcers

ulcers spread in her throat to the almost total loss of the velum pendulum palati: I then applied mercurial plasters to the throat outwardly, gave her a decoction of guaiacum for her constant drink, and calomel inwardly; but all to so little purpose, that in the sixth month I was obliged to have recourse to a mercurial friction, which I persisted in to the day of her delivery, as in all that time I was able only to check the disease, not to cure it. In her lying-in, she had severe cholics and fits of looseness, probably the effects of the method she had pursued. During her last course, and after her lying-in, besides the outward and inward use of mercury, she had drank above an hundred quarts of the decoction of guaiacum, strong and weak together. In July 1753, I proposed to her the decoction of sarsaparilla: at that time her pains were so severe, that she had

had not slept, for several months, an hour at a time; her body was become a mere skeleton; the ulcers in her throat were so nauseous, and her palate was so decayed, that she was become intolerable to herself, and greatly dispirited. The night after drinking the first bottle, she slept several hours, and so continued to do every night afterwards without interruption: in twenty days her head-aches and nocturnal pains entirely left her: in seven days more her throat was quite well; she recovered her speech; and, by the use of thirty seven quarts of the decoction, she was restored to perfect health, strength, and spirits; her breasts becoming plump and full, as usual; and to the day of writing this (September 1754) she still enjoys an uninterrupted state of health.

Q   CASE

CASE II.

That same summer, a watchmaker of a scorbutic habit of body, with spungy gums, who had been salivated three different times, and had used great variety of alteratives, and decoctions of guaiacum without measure, applied to me. He all that time had foul sores in the tonsils, numberless blotches dry and moist on his body, and chancres on his penis, attended with a sort of gleet: these were all his venereal symptoms. I put him upon the use of the decoction of sarsaparilla, to the quantity of a quart daily. After he had taken it fifty six days, all the symptoms left him; but the parts where the chancres had been, though skinned over, continued red, oozing at times a sort of ichor. For these, and now and then a little sort of gleeting from

the

the urethra, I have tried every thing I could think of, but all to little or no effect. Dr. Barry's alterative pills, composed of turpeth mineral, pil. ex duobus, and camphire, have done most apparent service.†

CASE III.

Some weeks after this, a jeweller, who had contracted a clap, for which he had been unsuccessfully treated, applied to me for a cure: when I saw him he had chancres, and verrucæ mixed all round the corona glandis and behind it, but no other venereal complaint. He drank about fifty bottles of the decoction of sarsaparilla; but till he had rubbed on six ounces of mercurial ointment, the chancres were not entirely healed; the last of which he used after he had omitted

† See Medical Essays.

ted the decoction some time: nay, the verrucæ still remained, but were immediately removed by the common caustic. I would remark, by the bye, that in cases of venereal warts, where the infection seems to have been entirely subdued, the common caustic is the only application that I have used with certain success. I would therefore recommend it as the most efficacious in such cases. It is worthy of notice, that warts are among the most obstinate symptoms of the venereal disease; that they require an inunction well followed out; that if, when the common caustic has eaten them down, they shoot again, the antivenereal regimen must, after a proper interval, be repeated, or the patient remain poxed.

CASE IV.

Much about the same time, a grenadier of the third regiment of foot guards, on whom

whom I had tried mercurial alteratives, and decoctions of guaiacum, after having first attempted a cure by a salivation, was put upon the decoction of sarsaparilla. At the time he began to take it, he had ill-digested buboes, chancres on his penis, foul ulcers in the tonsils and velum pendulum palati, as well as on the back part of the pharynx, and universal pains. He was unable to move his legs and arms, and had large black and mortified blotches and sloughs, some of them as large as a half crown piece, on his shoulders and back. By the use of this decoction for fifteen days, and two bleedings (which some feverish symptoms seemed to indicate) every one of the above complaints was removed, and he left the hospital apparently cured : but whether it was owing to his not having persisted long enough in the use of it, or to some other cause, in two or three weeks he came

came back to the hofpital with a fore throat, and complaining of his pains; when I put him a fecond time on the ufe of the decoction: though his throat grew better foon, yet the pains did not entirely go off; fometimes an arm, and at other times the leg and thigh, continuing in pain. During this fecond trial he drank twenty five bottles of the decoction. I then attempted the cure by mercurial pills, and a decoction of guaiacum, rubbing in now and then fome mercurial ointment; after which I fent him to country quarters, for the benefit of the air: but this not anfwering, he returned to the hofpital a third time, when his throat, and the back part of his pharynx, were much ulcerated; he was greatly emaciated; had a cough, night fweats, and gummatous fwellings on the top of his fhoulder, and on the wrifts: he then took a box of an alterative mercurial

pill

pill among other things, but all to no purpose; so that he repeated the decoction of sarsaparilla for the third time, and drank thirty nine bottles more; upon which his throat grew well; the pains and swellings were considerably diminished, and indeed so far, that there were scarce any remains of either, but about his knees. Soon after this he was discharged the regiment, being reckoned unfit for the service; and he returned to his native place, without giving the medicine a further trial, though he was pressed to do it. I have often blamed myself for not prosecuting the experiment further, in so remarkable a case, where, upon every fresh trial, the good effects were so manifest, and, if longer persisted in, might have produced a complete cure. Dr. Clephane and Dr. Pringle saw the progress of this patient's disease, both at the worst, and when the sarsaparilla did such service.

CASE V.

An oilman, who had gone through a mercurial courfe for a chancre on the glans penis, applied to me for advice, having at that time violent pain over all his body, efpecially fuch head-aches and continual watchings as rendered his life intolerable: he was unable to ftand upright, or to have any of his limbs moved; when I put him under a courfe of the farfaparilla decoction: the firft bottle of it compofed him to fleep the whole night, though for three months paft he had not flept one hour at a time; and he was thereby fo much relieved from his pains, and incapacity to move, that he foon was able to walk to me every day afterwards for his quart of decoction, and by thirty-fix bottles of it was perfectly cured: he ufed no other medicine or application,
except

except that during the courſe of the decoction he wore a ſlip of mercurial plaſter on the ſcar where the chancre had been.

CASE VI.

A widow lady, three months after her huſband's death, conſulted me about her health: ſhe complained of violent headaches, which had for ſome months paſt prevented her reſt, and of ſome hard and dry lumps which ſhe had perceived a few days before on the labia pudendi: her whole body was covered with large hard ſpots or blotches, of a browniſh red colour, but not attended with ſcurf or ſcales, excepting two that were on her leg. From theſe ſymptoms, and the account ſhe gave me of her huſband, I could not doubt of the nature of her diſeaſe: the ſcorbutic appearance of her gums, and her delicate

habit

habit of body, determined me to attempt the cure without a mercurial falivation, having for fome years paſt obſerved the very bad effects it is apt to produce on ſcorbutic habits, attended with ſpungy gums. By the uſe of forty bottles of the decoction, all the former ſymptoms left her, except the two large blotches on her leg: but ſhe then ſhewed me a chancre, large and hard, on the infide of the nymphæ, which ſhe had perceived only for two or three days, and which difcharged matter plentifully: I was thereupon forced to have immediate recourſe to a mercurial friction, as the weak ſtate of her ſtomach forbad the internal uſe of mercury. By perfifting fix weeks in this courſe, though I could only rub in a little ointment at a time, and even that frequently at the hazard of her fainting away, ſhe recovered a perfect ſtate of health. During the uſe of the decoction ſhe abſtained both from wine and

and meat, yet her ſtrength kept up well; but in the mercurial courſe it was found neceſſary to allow her wine and fleſh meats to ſupport her.

CASE VII.

In April laſt, a married lady from the country gave me the following hiſtory of her caſe.

In the fourth month of her pregnancy, ſhe had obſerved a number of little pimples break out on her face, which ſoon after grew ſcaly, increaſing every day in ſize and hardneſs: in her fifth month, her ſleep left her, ſhe was tortured with moſt violent head-aches, and nocturnal pains in her bones, particularly in one of her legs, where ſhe felt a hardneſs lying looſe under the ſkin, upon the ſhin bone, of the ſize of a horſe bean: ſhe likewiſe became very dull of hearing, but had no ſymptoms of the difease about the pudenda. In the eighth month, she was delivered of a weakly child, which, as she expressed it, was born without skin. The above named symptoms continued increasing till the end of the second month after her lying-in, at which time she applied to me for advice: after purging her gently with salts and manna, I gave her the decoction in the usual dose; but as I durst not, in such a case, trust entirely to it, I now and then used the mercurial ointment, to the quantity of half an ounce of quick-silver in the whole; and by the end of the month all her complaints left her, except the dullness of hearing, which still continues in some degree.

This is the only instance in which I confined any patient to their bed or flannels, or to a strict regimen during the use of the decoction, and the only instance where the nocturnal pains were not quite

removed

removed by a few doses of the sarsaparilla. I should likewise note, that I cut out the small gummatous tumour with a knife, while she was using the sarsaparilla.

CASE VIII.

A wine-merchant's servant in the Strand had, for twelve months and upwards, chancres on his penis; for which he was put under, and persisted in, a mercurial course by unction for four months, the mercury seldom affecting his mouth to any degree. As his being much abroad exposed him to catch frequent colds, he was seized with rheumatic pains all over him, which at first were alleviated by repeated bleedings, but grew so bad at last, that he almost entirely lost the use of his limbs, though he tried various medicines for them. He continued in this state till we put him on a decoction of sarsaparilla;
by

by forty four bottles of which he recovered his former state of health, without any confinement or regimen; though he was often abroad, exposed to the cold and wet, during the time of his drinking the decoction, which was in the month of November.

CASE IX.

An officer's servant in the guards had two buboes forming in his groins, without any other symptom of the pox, when he applied to me. As he was then under a necessity of going abroad, I applied mercurial plasters to his buboes, and supplied him with ointment sufficient to secure his health by repeated unctions. Finding his throat affected, he applied for advice when in Germany, but did not persist in the mercurial unction; by which neglect he
returned

returned to London with a deep and foul ulcer in the back part of his throat.

I then anointed him regularly, and gave him strong decoctions of guaiacum to the quantity of thirty bottles and upwards; by which the ulcer in his throat was healed, and he was apparently well: six weeks after, he was seized with a deep-seated pain in his cheek bone, and a swelling upon it, which in fourteen days brought on sickness, vomiting, a total loss of appetite, and night sweats, which emaciated him greatly. I laid the bone of his cheek bare, and found that it was carious, but it had no marks of being likely soon to exfoliate. I then put him on the decoction of sarsaparilla, of which he drank forty bottles: in six days after he began the use of it, his appetite returned, his sickness went off, his sweats ceased, and by the end of the course he was become fleshy, and as fresh coloured as usual; some weeks after which, there came out an exfoliation of the size of a silver groat, and of a considerable thickness. This person is now in perfect health.

CASE X.

Mrs. Gordon in Chandos-street, when she applied to me, told me, that in her first husband's time she had sores in her legs, which were suddenly dried up; and that she found no bad consequence from them, till she had lived with her second husband four or five years, and had had two fine children by him, apparently very healthy; when she was taken with violent pains in her head, nose, and face, for which she tried various medicines, and among other courses was salivated regularly, and afterwards used an application of Mr. Plunkett's; during which

courses

courses she lost the bones of her nose. She had likewise applied afterwards at an hospital for advice, where she was put under a course of Dog and Duck water, and such diet as was judged proper in cases that seemed cancerous. When she applied to me, I understood, by the history of her case, that it was a venereal one, contracted from her first husband, but that it had appeared first in her head, and never in her pudenda: I put her upon a course of the sarsaparilla, desiring her at the same time to wash the sores of her face with some of the decoction, and then to cover them with dry lint. These sores had been of six months standing, when I saw her first; and the nose not only was become quite flat, with a foul sore upon it, but the frontal bone, the temporal bone, the orbital bone of the right eye, and the upper maxillary bone, were bare in several places. When in this condition, Dr. Clephane vifited her with me, and Mr. John Hunter had feen her a few weeks before. By the ufe of the decoction for fifty days, inwardly and outwardly applied, as before mentioned, all the fores healed up, fome of the bones threw off exfoliations, others of them covered over without any fenfible exfoliation, and fhe recovered her health perfectly, with only the lofs of the bones of her nofe, and a few fcars on her face.

CASE XI.

Jamefon, a foldier of the third regiment, recovered, by thirty nine bottles of a weaker decoction of farfaparilla, of pocky pains; for which, and fome other venereal complaints, he had been falivated thrice, kept his bed in the hofpital for two hundred and thirty days and upwards,

wards, was emaciated greatly, and had tried in vain all forts of antivenereal, antiscorbutic, or antirheumatic medicines.

N. B. After several months this patient applied to me again, complaining of fresh ulcers in his throat, and, as he says, without having catched a fresh infection. But what is very remarkable in this instance is, that his relapse was probably owing to his having used only the small decoction, or rather what may be called the second decoction.

CASE XII.

A gentleman's servant in St. James's place, who had spurious buboes for six months, for which he went through two regular courses by unction, during his first course had a partial suppuration from one of them, continued to have pain in that, and a large tumour of the size of a hen's egg remained, which would not give way to any application, and at the same time lay so deep, and was so much engaged with the iliac artery, as to prevent our destroying it by caustic. Ten bottles of the decoction removed it without suppuration, and he drank twenty four more for security's sake.

CASE XIII.

The husband of the lady mentioned in Case VII. was, at the same time with her, put under a mercurial course for chancres all round the glans penis, blotches on the scrotum and thighs, ragged sores about his anus, and foul ulcers in his throat. After using about eight ounces of mercurial ointment, and salivating plentifully, for six weeks, all his complaints left him, except those ragged sores about his anus, which remained as obstinate

ſtinate as ever, though the mercurial ointment had been rubbed on them alſo about the end of the courſe, and though he had been ſweated very ſufficiently by fourteen quart bottles of the ſtrong decoction of guaiacum; but they gave way in a few days to the decoction of ſarſaparilla.*

I ſhall therefore juſt offer the reſult of my experience, in relation to the ſarſaparilla, by deducing from theſe, and above as many more caſes, in which I have tried it, a few remarks, tending to ſhew when it will cure, and when it will fail.

REMARK I.

It will commonly relieve, in a very ſhort ſpace of time, venereal head-aches and nocturnal pains; and, if perſiſted in, I believe, will always cure.

---

* See a note from Fallopius, page 141, which relates particularly to this ſymptom.

REMARK II.

In emaciated or confumptive habits, from a venereal caufe, it is the greateft reftorer of appetite, flefh, colour, ftrength, and vigour, that I know of.

REMARK III.

When the throat, nofe, palate, or the fpungy bones in general, are affected with a flough or caries, it will commonly complete the cure, if perfevered in long enough, and providing a mercurial courfe, I mean by unction, has preceded the ufe of the farfaparilla. It is precifely in fuch cafes, where the wonder-working powers of farfa are not only abfolutely neceffary for the cure, but produce a perfect one.

REMARK IV.

When the body is covered with dry blotches, or moift fores (ftill fuppofing the caufe venereal) it will greatly promote the

the cure, nay, often complete it; but, without the affiftance of mercury, there will be danger of a relapfe.

REMARK V.

In fimple chancres it will do little fervice; but if it is given in cafes where the chancres or buboes will not heal or diffolve, after the ufe of mercurial unction, it will often cure, and always do manifeft fervice.

REMARK VI.

It will oftentimes anfwer, and that fpeedily, without fweating, confinement, or any very ftrict regimen, at all feafons of the year, where mercurial unctions, and long continued courfes of ftrong decoctions of guaiacum, either by itfelf fimply, or compounded with a fmall proportion of our farfaparilla, have failed. Of this I could produce feveral other proofs, befides the above hiftories.

REMARK VII.

It would seem probable, from any observations I have yet been able to make, *that the sarsaparilla root is only to be depended on in venereal cases where mercury has failed, at least has preceded the use of the decoction, or when it is combined with it; and therefore is not to be trusted to alone, unless in such circumstances:* and this is agreeable to the well known effects of that medicine, the reputation of which, in inveterate venereal cases, first put me on making this enquiry.

REMARK VIII.

Mercury alone will in general cure most venereal complaints; the sarsaparilla will perhaps always cure what resists the power of mercury: it is therefore probable, that we may find in mercury and sarsaparilla, pro-
perty

perly combined, a certain cure for every case that can be called venereal.

Let us now see,

I. What this medicine is.

II. Whence it came.

III. What reputation it had at first.

IV. If the esteem it acquired in Europe was founded on accurate observations of its effects.

V. How it lost it again, and has been but little used till very lately: and,

VI. How it ought to be prepared and given.

It is doubted by botanical writers, whether it was known to Theophrastus and Diascorides; but if it is of the same genus with our smilax aspera, which both from its appearance and virtues I am apt to believe it is, this cannot remain doubtful, since the first has described the plant, and the second mentions its virtues as an alexipharmic.

T   Fallopius

Fallopius used the smilax aspera, which he found growing near Pisa, and cured many with it;* nay, alledges that the virtues of the European are more powerful than those of the Indian, ascribing their external difference to the different soils in which they grow. And Carolus Musitanus asserts, that the smilax aspera, which grows plentifully in Italy, under the name of the salsa paesana, only differs in price from that of Peru; but that the taste, bark, pith, and virtues, are stronger and more vegete in the European than in the Indian sort.†

Prosper Alpinus has put it beyond all doubt, by the appearance of the smilax aspera, which he found in soft grounds, in the island of Zant, (Zacynthus) that Europe,

---

* Loco sarsaparillæ semper cum felici successu. *Fallopii tractatus de morbo Gallico, caput* 63.

† Carol. Musitanus de lue venerea. lib. iii. cap. 1. in Sarsaparillam.

Europe, and the Grecian iſlands in particular, furniſh the true farſaparilla, or ſmilax aſpera, (Peruviana dicta) of C. B.*

The medicine which is the ſubject of our preſent enquiry, and is now to be found in every druggiſt's ſhop, is the root of the ſmilax aſpera Peruviana of Caſpar Bauhin. It is brought to us from Peru, Hiſpaniola, and the Brazils.

Monardes tells us, that the Indians, when they begin to uſe it, taſte nothing but the decoction and its mucilage (lentorem) for the firſt three days, and afterwards only almonds, raiſins, and bread, during the thirty days courſe of it.

The method of preparing it by the Spaniards and Indians of South America, is as follows: They macerate an ounce of the root in almoſt four pints, or pounds, of water, for twenty four hours, and boil it

---

* Proſper. Alpin. de plant. Ægypt. c. 43.

it away to one half. They give of the expressed decoction half a pint twice a day, four hours before their meals, in bed, covered with clothes, where they sweat two hours, mixing a sufficient quantity of the fine powder of the root with each dose of the decoction. They purge them every tenth day.

The Spaniards first brought it into Europe, towards the middle of the sixteenth century.

Franciscus Ximenes, in his annotations to Margravius's natural history of the Brazils, talks of its speedy and powerful effects in the cure of the lues venerea, given in simple decoction.†

Vidus Vidius, about the year 1550, gives

---

† Cujus decocto simplici ad luem veneream, præsertim non inveteratam, nihil præstantius, quippe quod observatâ diætâ, paucis intermissis diebus, a turpi et fœdo malo ægros vindicat. *Margravius in historia naturali Brasil. de Sarsaparilla.*

gives it the third place among antivenereal decoctions. §

Trincavellius prefers it to guaiacum as an attenuant, and makes mention of it as a resolver of hard tumors. ||

‡ Gabriel Fallopius seems to have known more of the virtues of the sarsaparilla than most of his predecessors or successors, if we except Trajanus Petronius alone, of whom afterwards.

In

---

§ Vidus Vidius, in morbo Gallico, de Sarsaparilla.

|| Vim majorem habet attenuandi & digerendi quam guaiaci decoctum, si duros & quasi tophosos tumores in internodiis articulorum concretos digerere, & quasi atterere potest, ut quotidie videmus. *Trincavell. Consil.* 50.

‡ Recenseamus experimentum cui nolunt credere pertinaces. Diascorides dicit habere vim antidoti in morbis contagiosis, & connumerat grana & folia inter ea medicamenta quæ venenis exhibentur; ideo regium est auxilium & antidotum ad fugandam luem veneream. Et hac ratione ego fido magis salsæ quàm ligno guaiaci: imbecillior est certè ligno; habet tamen ipsa nobiles vires, quibus superat guaiacum; et est, quòd si,

post

In the Venetian edition of Fallopius * mention is made of this decoction not keeping above five or six days. I never could keep it above three, even in a cellar: no author besides Floyer, that I know of, takes the least notice of this. I believe it has been owing to their not attending to such a circumstance, that it

post superatum Gallicum, restant ulcera rhagadia circa sedem, duplo citiùs sanat hæc quàm lignum Indicum. Erat scholaris Papiensis qui tophis osseis & lapideis laborabat circa pedes & tibias: ego brevi discussos vidi ope salsæparillæ, & prima vice usus sum hâc in milite Lucensi qui dicebatur (*Il Capitan Capm*) hic habebat in capite tumores & gummata, quæ per decem dies evanuerant omnia: cum ergo in Gallico adsunt ulcera, ad hoc medicamentum confugio tanquam ad certissimum auxilium: si non facit prima dieta, faciet saltem secunda & tertia. Salsa est regina in hoc, quia discutit tophos quodam quasi miraculo. Decoctum salsæ semper agit omnibus temporibus: decoctum guaiaci non agit tempestate hiemali. *Fallop. tractat. de morb. Gallic.*, cap. 63, & 95. c. 95.

* Durat decoctum salsæ, si non sit tempus calidissimum, quinque vel sex diebus ad summum. *Vide Fallop. vol. 2. pa.* 166. *Edit. Venet.* 1651.

it was supposed to hurt the stomach, which I never knew it once do, if given alone, and in two days after it had been boiled in the way I propose it to be done.

Massarias prefers it to the guaiacum for dispatch, agreeableness, and virtues. ‡

Cæsalpinus says it hurts the stomach, but resolves gummatous swellings; and prefers the outer bark of the root. †

Varandæus says it quiets pains in the joints. §

Thomas

‡ Tumores, gummata, pustulas, ulcera, & omnia symptomata Gallica, longè faciliùs et breviore tempore, ex decocto Sarsaparillæ, mitigari & deleri, quàm ligni decocto. *Massarias practic. medic. p. 905.*

† Ventriculo noxia est, sed facit magis ad gummositates. *Cæsalpin. artis medicæ lib. 4. de morbo Gallico.*

§ Sarsaparillam habere proprietatem ad dolores artuum sedandos. *Varandæi de lui venerea.*

Thomas Rudius acknowledges that it is stronger in its virtues than guaiacum, but will not allow it to cure the disease alone radically. *

Nicolaus Massa, who has given us many formulæ of the stronger decoctions of sarsaparilla, says, that in strength it equals the guaiacum wood in the cure of the disease. †

Alexander Trajanus Petronius also compares

---

* Longè meliùs dolores tum Gallicos tum alios demulcere quàm guaiacum; sed Gallicum virus, nisi admodum exiguum, & in corpore recenter contractum sit, per seipsum profligare & extirpare impotentem esse: ideoque ipsum non verum & legitimum luis venereæ bezoarticum medicamentum esse. *Rudii Lib.* iv. *c.* 2. *de morbo Gallico.*

† Sanat tumores duros, et ulcera antiqua Gallici morbi, & omnia vitia & mala, in quâcunque corporis parte, quæ in morbo Gallico accidere consuevêre, & quæ solent sanari ligni Indici decoctione bibitâ, quoniam omnes ferè virtutes, quæ in ligno Indico sunt, in sarsa reperiuntur. *Nichol. Massa de morbo Gallico, cap.* 10.

pares its effects to those of guaiacum, and recommends it very strongly. †

We see therefore, that many of its virtues, in venereal cases, have been carefully noted by the Europeans; but that they were

† Prodest decoctum sarsæ, quemadmodum guaiaci dococtum, omnibus lue Gallicâ inquinatis; sed quanto quàm illud tenuiorum partium est, tanto celeriùs auxiliatur, potissimùm verò his, quibus caput insigniter dolet, postquam guaiaci decoctum ante exhibitum aut parum aut nihil contulit: adde etiam, ut cuidam placet, ulcera, et circa sedem rhagadia, multo celeriùs quam decoctum guaiaci curare, & gummationes dissolvere, consuevit. Sarsaparilla pollet adversus eum qui suâ natura mitis est, aut incipit, aut inclinat, aut si quidem sævus fuerit, aliis tamen remediis attritus atque subactus, hominem adhuc infestat. Hinc certè vim magnam in morbum Gallicum habere sarsaparilla creditur, utpote quem guaiacum non sanârit, hæc postea sanat: sanat enim immanem, quem guaiacum, aut siquid hujusmodi antea mutavit, mitigavit atque dissolvit; non sanat verò *si statim ab initio contra illum* sumatur: quocirca sarsæ decoctum luem quidem Gallicam evertit; sed quia debiles sunt ejus vires, non nisi mitem, aut incipientem, aut declinantem, aut omnino si sæva fuerit postquam aliis remediis ante demissa devictaque sit, evertit. *Alex. Trajani Petronii lib.* v. *cap.* 2, & 4.

were not thoroughly acquainted with them all: they did not determine its powers of extirpating the difeafe though ever fo intimately mixed with the habit, and which had efcaped the virtues of mercury in every fhape: they were ignorant of its curing the difeafe without confinement, (*Ceftoni alone excepted) fweating, or a regimen: though they knew that it made the fymptoms difappear, they were ignorant how to prevent their return: though they gave ftrong decoctions ‡ of farfaparilla, yet they all erred in macerating it fo long in the water, before they boiled it; which fpoils it for ufe after forty eight hours. Nor did they determine accurately the cafes in which it might be depended on, and what proportion of the root would anfwer. Hence it is perhaps, that

we

---

* *Cefton.* vide *la Galleria di Minerv.* tom. vi. *part* 3; and there, *Lettera fcritta dall Signore Ceftoni.*

‡ *Nicolaus Maffa de morbo Gallico, cap.* 11.

we find them complaining that it hurt the ſtomach, though it is now certainly known that, if properly prepared, it re-ſtores the appetite and digeſtion even where the patient becomes hectic, from a venereal cauſe, unleſs perſevered in beyond two dozen of quarts at one courſe; for we have ſeen inſtances in which a ſecond was neceſſary. They were but little acquainted with its uſe in venereal pains, and where the bones are affected; and yet it is preciſely in ſuch caſes that it ſeems to ſhew its greateſt efficacy.*

Thus it fell into diſrepute, and by degrees

* It were to be wiſhed, that ſome of thoſe benevolent ſpirits with which this bleſs'd country (*bona ſi ſua nôrint*) abounds, would ſet on foot a ſubſcription, in the hoſpitals where the diſeaſe in queſtion is peculiarly cared for, to purchaſe enough of this moſt valuable root, to allow of its ſtrong decoction being given in *all* caſes where the throat, noſe, or bones are affected; as I will be bold to affirm, that in ſuch caſes, without its aſſiſtance, mercury alone, whether given inwardly or applied outwardly, will very ſeldom *eſtabliſh* a cure.

grees was almoſt forgotten, infomuch that of late fome of our greateſt maſters in medicine have aſſerted that its decoction is no better than barley water.

I would fay therefore, that in this iſland, notwithſtanding the inconſtancy of the climate, and irregularity of living, it will produce the effects that I have hinted at above in this enquiry, if prepared and given in the following manner.

To three ounces of the farfaparilla root, as freſh as it can be procured, not fpoiled with age, worms, fea water or moiſture, add three quarts of river water, and bring it to boil immediately in an open veſſel, (I always ordered a copper one) and let it boil away to two pints of the ſtrained liquor, that is, to about two pounds avoirdupoife. I fometimes add a little liquorice root, to make it more palatable. This quantity I give at two or three doſes, either warm or cold, as it is

moſt

moſt agreeable, every twenty four hours. Every other day it muſt be made freſh, and what is not uſed the day it is boiled, muſt be kept in a cold cellar. I have always recommended abſtemious living, particularly with regard to wine.

With relation to this diſeaſe in children, it may not be from the purpoſe to obſerve, that, on the credit of Harris de Lue Venerea, I ſeveral years ago gave it in powder, and in decoction at the ſame time: but hitherto I cannot boaſt of its having radically cured the complaint, probably becauſe mercury had not been uſed before, or becauſe the children did not perſiſt long enough in the uſe of it.*

I have

---

* I have, ſince the above was written, learned from more experience, that the youngeſt children may have the diſeaſe rooted out by mercurial frictions, if uſed *very* gently, and continued for a *long* time, according to the ſtrength of the patient.

I have some reason to believe, but have not hitherto had experience sufficient to determine, that those rheumatic complaints (I call them so because they appear as such) which are so common, and so obstinate, after a mercurial course, may be cured by strong decoctions of sarsaparilla. I give this hint, because there are few diseases that resist more the power of medicine than this; so obstinate indeed it is, that oftentimes it will not yield to a second mercurial unction.

I shall conclude with observing, that the root consists of two parts; the first, which is thick, dry, hard, and woody; and the other, which Astruc calls the flagellæ, which grow out of the thick part to a great length, and are soft, more succulent, and mucilaginous. The former in decoction is rather disagreeable; the latter not offensive, and is the part I would be understood to mean in this paper; although

I have

I have reason, from some trials, to believe that the woody part is not inferior in virtue, where the stomach will bear it: perhaps too it might be usefully combined with the other; but this I must leave to be determined by future experiment.

THE END.

N. B. Since the Note on the swelled testicle was printed, (p. 44). I have found, in Dr. Layard's Essay on the Bite of a Mad Dog, published in 1762, mention made of the Mumps, with the Hernia Humoralis, as a symptom, having been endemical among the Essex militia quartered in the town of Huntingdon, in the months of February, March, and April, 1760.

www.ingramcontent.com/pod-product-compliance
Lightning Source LLC
Chambersburg PA
CBHW030435190426
43202CB00036B/896